"A stimulating book that effectively tells the story of psycho-nutrition as we now understand it."
—*Human Behavior*

PSYCHO-NUTRITION

The essential guide to better emotional health. Learn the facts about:

- COMMON NEUROSES—How nutritional deficiencies contribute to the symptoms of everyday disorders, as well as psychoses and schizophrenia.

- ALLERGIES—How this common problem can produce the symptoms of hyperactivity, paranoia, neuroses, and other psychological disturbances.

- HYPOGLYCEMIA—How this "hidden" disease can cause symptoms of acute psychosis, and how it can be controlled with a simple diet plan.

- ORTHOMOLECULAR THERAPY—The megavitamin treatment that relieves or cures psychological symptoms by treating their biological causes.

Discover the emotionally healing powers of vitamins and minerals. Forge a happier, healthy life through . . . PSYCHO-NUTRITION

CARLTON FREDERICKS, Ph.D.

PSYCHO-NUTRITION

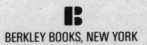

BERKLEY BOOKS, NEW YORK

This Berkley book contains the complete
text of the original edition.
It has been completely reset in a typeface
designed for easy reading and was printed
from new film.

PSYCHO-NUTRITION

A Berkley Book/published by arrangement with
G. P. Putnam's Sons

PRINTING HISTORY
Perigee Books edition published 1982
Berkley edition/September 1988

ISBN: 0-425-11055-9

A BERKLEY BOOK ® TM 757,375
Berkley Books are published by The Berkley Publishing Group,
200 Madison Avenue, New York, New York 10016.
The name ''BERKLEY'' and the ''B'' logo
are trademarks belonging to Berkley Publishing Corporation.

PRINTED IN THE UNITED STATES OF AMERICA

10 9 8 7 6 5 4 3 2 1

To an extraordinary and multifaceted man, who had daughters and their husbands, a son, grandchildren, and great-grandchildren, and was a father to us all. We loved Leon Schachter, and we miss him.

CARLTON FREDERICKS

An Acknowledgment

I HAVE WATCHED the tragedies of emotional disorder and mental disease in friends, in radio listeners, in readers of my books, in young students in the university classes I teach, and in a beloved member of my own family. I know firsthand the impact on a family of the mental sickness of a member. I have watched with anguish and frustration the attempts at suicide so frequent in the schizophrenias. I know to what extent the psychotropic drugs mask or quiet the symptoms, what residual disease hides behind the fragile defenses built by unphysiological medication, and at what prices in dangerous side reactions these tenuous gains are achieved. I am therefore sensitively aware of the sterility of conventional psychiatric therapies in coping with the psychoses, and the blindness of the profession to the influence of body on mind. That sterility is as complete as the implacable resistance of the profession to the concept that mental disorder is a reflection of biochemical chaos—a concept explicit in *orthomolecular*—"the right molecule"—therapies.

No one knows better than I that orthomolecular psychiatry is no panacea. I have witnessed some of its failures, but I have also seen its triumphs, and I know that it often offers a new level of hope from a new kind of help for the psychotic, the neurotic, the brain-damaged, the autistic, the retarded, and the slow learner. Even more exciting is the challenge it offers in potential improvement of the *normal*. These are my reasons for wishing to acknowledge the contributions of the pioneers in the biochemical-nutritional approach to the problems of mental and emotional dysfunction. I am grateful (as you one day may be) for what we have learned from Dr. Linus Pauling, Dr. Bernard Rimland, Dr. H. L. Newbold, Dr. William Philpott, Dr. Marshall Mandell, Dr. Abram Hoffer, Dr. Humphrey Osmund, Dr. Carl Pfeiffer, Dr. Allan Cott, Dr. David Hawkins, Dr. Paul Dunn, Dr. Ray Wunderlich, and many others, too numerous to name, of my friends and colleagues in the International Academy of Preventive Medicine, the Academy of Orthomolecular Psychiatry, the International Academy of Metabology, and the International College of Applied Nutrition.

These professional men and these societies form the advance guard—in science, always the target for severe and often irrational hostility—in the battle against the molecules of madness. The term is carefully chosen, for whether the psychosis is gene-dictated, or the price of intolerable strain, or the direct result of a derangement of the exquisitely concatenated chemistries of the brain and nervous system, in the end, the mental sickness is a molecular disease, or it is not a disease at all.

Contents

Foreword

DR. I. N. KUGELMASS, distinguished physician, biochemist, hematologist, and nutritionist, views us as two systems which transform raw materials, supplied by the environment, in "serviceable ways."

Physiologically, body chemistry elaborates Nature's materials into physiochemical compounds intended precisely to meet the needs of the body machine, its bone, muscle, glands, tissue, blood vessels, and cells. This is physiometabolism.

The other system is psychometabolism. Its basic material is subjective experience; its product is, hopefully, psychosocially acceptable organization of feeling and thought.

"Psycho-nutrition" is a wedding of these concepts, for we are and we think and we feel and function and are maintained with what we eat. If our nutrition—always a compromise falling short of the optimal—in any way fails us, what we are, think, and feel will change; and these changes will feed back to and alter psychometabolism. Conversely, when nutritional deficits are repaired—which may require heroic amounts of nutrients usually needed in much smaller maintenance quantities—the responses in terms of more socially acceptable feeling and thought may (and often do) make the difference between being a dweller within the scene and being an outcast on its fringe or a cipher in its mental institutions. So it is that psycho-nutrition is more than a new approach to the problems of the neurotic, the schizophrenic, the alcoholic, and the withdrawn, hyperactive, autistic, slow learner, or minimally brain-damaged, for—excitingly—it also extends to *normal* children and adults a means, too long neglected, of reaching potentials they never knew they had.

PART I

·1·

It's Not All in Your Mind

SHE WAS ONLY eleven when she first experienced the mental and physical disturbances which psychiatrists found unresponsive to all their traditional treatments. She was obviously schizophrenic, with many of the distortions of perception which are characteristic of that group of disorders. Living in an unreal world, from which ultimately she could not return, tortured with paranoid delusions, she became depressed to the point of a suicide attempt before she reached puberty. Amnesia developed—she could not, for instance, remember trying to hang herself; severe convulsions began, which were not relieved by the usual anti-epilepsy medications. By the time she was fifteen, she was a veteran of years of psychotherapy, group therapy, shock treatment, and hundreds of prescriptions for psychotropic drugs, ranging from tranquilizers to antidepressants.

It was at fifteen that she had her first encounter with an orthomolecular psychiatrist. The term means "the right molecules." It reflects a concept in psychology which is not new—Freud himself thought that the chemistry of the brain is disturbed in "mental" disorders—but one which only recently has been accepted and applied effectively by a growing number of practitioners. Biochemical examination of the girl revealed inadequate production of three enzymes critical to the normal chemistry of the brain. One of these enzymes depends upon a vitamin, the other two on "trace" minerals,

3

so called because the quantities ordinarily needed by the body are minute. Generous doses of these nutrients were given. The convulsions stopped, the amnesia disappeared, and she returned to the world of reality, minus her depression and her delusions of persecution. She is normal, and will remain so, as long as she takes her daily ration of the critical vitamin and the two trace minerals.

Her story is told in detail in Chapter Three. I touch upon it here because it is such a good example of a victory of orthomolecular psychiatry in one of a group of diseases which have shown so little response to psychotherapy, tranquilizers, and other conventional treatments that schizophrenias for years have filled more hospital beds than any other disease.

It is predictable that the old guard in psychiatry and psychology would be up in arms against the basic concepts of orthomolecular medicine applied to "mental" and "emotional" disorders. The psychoanalyst by the very nature of his training cannot accept the proposition that thinking and perceptions are biological functions of the brain as digestion is of the stomach; and that both may be altered biochemically. Conversely, responses like those of the little girl may easily persuade orthomolecular psychiatrists to forget that those tortured by deranged chemistry of the brain may also be victims of purely emotional and mental stresses, which likewise plead for treatment by the orthodox means. This is to say that the woman who is paranoid because Vitamin B_{12} deficiency has attacked the very structure of her brain and nervous system may still have people who genuinely hate her. And, unless the orthomolecular psychiatrist is capable of very broad and flexible thinking, he may not perceive the need for conventional treatment of the patient to help compensate for the mental and emotional insults a psychotic endures in his years of suffering. Finally, orthodox psychiatry and orthomolecular psychiatrists may not appreciate the vicious circle which is so beautifully illustrated in the problem of hypoglycemia (low blood sugar), where tension and anxiety may trigger low blood sugar which in turn causes tension and anxiety.

I heard a classic exchange between an analyst and an orthomolecular psychiatrist. The analyst said: "You give these patients vitamins, minerals, hypoglycemia diets, chelating agents, tranquilizers, lithium, and sometimes, shock therapy—and you call that 'orthomolecular'?" To which the orthomolecular practitioner appropriately rejoined, "You give your patient lithium, psychoenergizers, antidepressants, psychotherapy, soothing baths, and sessions on the couch—and you call that 'psychiatric treatment'?"

One can understand that medicine has been particularly resistant to the introduction of new ideas. In fact, medical men are specifically trained to be extremely cautious in adopting innovation—the phrase goes: 'Be not the first to adopt the new, nor the last to cast the old aside." That leads to the sequence so aptly described by Montaigne: When first discovered, it is untrue. Twenty years later, it is true but not important. Thirty years more, and it is true and important, but it's fifty years old—we have something better now! Unfortunately, that cultural lag, if it is allowed to operate unhindered in the field of psychiatry, will keep those mental hospital beds filled for another half century, with patients who could have been—and weren't—helped. All this is by way of reminding the old guard in psychiatry that they are not speaking from a position of strength. They are not being asked to try a new modality to replace a tested, reliable, and productive one. Every mental hospital is an epitaph to the bankruptcy of conventional psychiatry—unless you wish to consider patients so heavily tranquilized that they are vegetables, no longer requiring straitjackets, to represent a therapeutic triumph.

The truth, of course, is not always found between two extremes, but in this case, it is. Certainly, schizophrenia is not based on too much or too little mother love, too dominant or too passive a father, or emotional deprivation in the formative years. Conversely, not all schizophrenics will be dramatically helped by doses of these vitamins or those minerals. However, the *total* failures reported in megavitamin treatments for schizophrenics usually derive from research which involves three fallacious assumptions. It is a fallacy to believe that schizophrenia is a single disease which can be treated in a single way, or for that matter with a single vitamin. Second, not all cases of a single type of schizophrenia will necessarily respond to a single type of treatment. Third, it is not possible to treat early, chronic, mild, and acute schizophrenias with a uniform therapeutic regime. The papers which report total lack of success with orthomolecular treatment of mental disease frequently reflect one or more of these fallacies. Among the fruits of the research of Dr. Abram Hoffer, a pioneer in orthomolecular psychiatry, was the realization that only very early and very mild schizophrenia is likely to respond to doses, however large, of one single B vitamin (niacin). Yet orthodox psychiatrists, in an effort to reject the orthomolecular concept, point to reports of complete therapeutic failure in the administration of this single vitamin to a large mental hospital population. By definition, such a population would be highly unlikely to include very early and very mild schizophrenics. In another example of gratuitous obstruction of progress, we see a paper in which an eminent psychiatric researcher also reports complete failure with megavitamin dosage in schizophrenia. Only the close and well-informed reader would realize that the scientist used one vitamin—in the wrong chemical form, in an inadequate dose, for an inadequate period of time—on a group of psychotics with very severe schizophrenia of so many years' duration that only some type of as yet undiscovered biological dynamite could possibly stir them.

Against such negative reports, we might contrast the experience of professional practitioners who *themselves* were schizophrenic, and who were rescued by megavitamin therapy and controlled diet. For those who will immediately object to "anecdotal science" let me anticipate by pointing out that the patients themselves were excellent observers, since one was a psychiatrist and the other a psychotherapist. The psychiatrist had diagnosed himself as suffering from a catatonic schizophrenia, replete with hallucinations and suicidal depressions. He was disorientated in time and place, but well aware that the hallucinations (which were all visual) were not real. He felt "vague and awful" fears, which he described as a "a vague feeling of something alive, waiting for the right moment to attack" him. He had physical sensations of pressure in his forehead and stomach, and the illusion that his stomach and bowels were "dead." When he closed his eyes, constant pictures in color crossed his field of vision. These ranged from the grotesque to the frankly obscene, but he was again aware that these were hallucinations of a disturbed mind. He further described other hallucinations as being exactly the same as those caused by doses of mescaline, a drug known to cause such symptoms. His sense of touch was so abnormally heightened that his fingers, he thought, could feel every individual thread in a fabric. He could not distinguish distances between near objects, and became, consequently, clumsy. Exactly as the phenomenon occurs with mescaline and marijuana, perception of time became distorted, with minutes seeming to be hours, and hours feeling like centuries. Often he stood, staring into blankness, waiting for the inevitable hideous faces to appear—a condition that sometimes, to him, represented a catatonic stupor.

He had so many physical symptoms that I shall not pause here to describe them, including episodes of acute shortness of breath, bringing with them acute terror of impending death, in paroxysms which increased in violence until he collapsed, like an exhausted stag at bay, on the floor or bed.

Hoffer, who reports this case, notes that one of the tranquilizers, a rather mild one, dramatically—but temporarily—terminated his symptoms. Dr. Hoffer prescribed, instead, a gram each of nicotinic acid (a B-complex vitamin) and ascorbic acid (Vitamin C) three times daily, together with a sugar-free diet. Three hours after the first dose, there was an abrupt and significant reduction of all his symptoms, and his fears and anxieties were replaced by internal peace as he realized that for the first time in many years he was on the way toward complete recovery. This prompt improvement continued and increased over the next forty-eight hours, and by the time that he returned to the psychiatrist's office—a period of not more than a month of treatment—he was free of all symptoms.

In the second case I mentioned above, a psychotherapist found herself catatonic—a prisoner within her own body. Her experience was to her as frightening as that of the psychiatrist whose history you have just read, and she, too, recognized what was happening. She developed most of the classical symptoms of schizophrenia: hearing voices, feeling suicidally depressed without cause, considering herself unworthy to live, and suffering from unprovoked anxieties and unjustified fears. Conventional psychiatric treatment not only did not help, but allowed the disease to worsen until, as she describes it, she consulted an orthomolecular psychiatrist, feeling herself to be at the end of her resources and prepared to destroy herself. Examination showed a severe hypoglycemia (which is present in perhaps 60 percent of schizophrenics), and the practitioner promptly placed her on a sugar-free diet, with megavitamin dosages. She is now in practice as a highly effective psychotherapist—the more so, perhaps, because ''she's been there.'' As a side note which is relevant in the light of preceding statements in this chapter, she is having her troubles with local medical men and psychiatrists because she insists on correction of the diets and the institution of vitamin and other nutritional treatments for the children with whom she works— and works very effectively, it should be noted.

Those who demand controlled research will object to case histories as being uncontrolled, which means that the power of suggestion has not been ruled out as a possible contribution to the recovery of the patients. But those who make this demand are the very ones who give a vitamin to a thousand schizophrenics, and report not *one* beneficial effect—leading to the obvious question: where was the power of suggestion in *that* experiment? Should not *one* case in the thousand show some improvement in response to the ritual, if the power of suggestion is indeed so viable a part of recovery from schizophrenia? The thesis should be oddly uncomfortable for psychoanalysts to pursue, considering that they are practitioners in a ''scientific'' discipline which has never proved its basic premises and which, by its very nature, can't really be subjected to "controlled research." The fact that is overlooked—ignorantly or deliberately—by those hypercritical of the orthomolecular approach is the large number of scientifically controlled investigations which *have* been conducted, which *are* in the scientific literature, and which *do* report significant research. The orthomolecular practitioner, certainly as well trained as his orthodox brethren, is aware that the "recovery rate" in schizophrenics can be a very deceptive index of the effectiveness of a treatment. Even the layman knows that mental patients who have been discharged from psychiatric hospitals have sometimes gone on to mass murder or suicide or both; and practitioners well know that a large percentage of those discharged from psychiatric institutions are likely to be re-admitted during succeeding months or years. One orthomolecular psychiatrist therefore measured the effectiveness of the biochemical treatment by comparing two groups of hospitalized schizophrenics. The first group was treated with a broad spectrum of the conventional therapies—drug, shock, and psychotherapy. The second group received orthomolecular treatment added to the conventional therapies. He then appraised (a) the percentage of patients who in a given time could be discharged from the hospital; and (b), more importantly, the percentage in both groups who had to return. Not only did the orthomolecular group show a significantly higher percentage of responses, but significantly fewer were re-admitted for renewed treatment.

As psychiatrists and psychologists may become obsessed with the concept that mental disease is purely mental, so must the orthomolecular practitioner resist the temptation to place overemphasis on a single biochemical approach to emotional and mental disorders. Low blood sugar is capable of mimicking neurosis and psychosis so faithfully that patients have wandered from physician to psychiatrist and back again for fifteen years before discovering that they were not "a little queer," crackpots, psychotics, neurotics, or "constitutional inadequates" but suffering with a physical disorder neatly epitomizing the impact of body on mind. Physicians who have watched the dramatic recovery of such patients may forgivably conclude that hypoglycemia is The Enemy. An orthomolecular psychiatrist who brings a little girl back to sanity with doses of zinc and manganese may understandably focus much of his attention on the minerals. The physician who has watched hyperactive children recover when food additives are removed from their diets will obviously devote much of his time to exploring the usefulness of additive-free food in the treatment of hyperactivity and, perhaps, other disorders once considered solely "mental" or "emotional."

One can understand, too, the preoccupation with food allergy which dominates the thinking of a psychiatrist who has watched patients recover from deep depression, merely by removal from the diet of a few offending foods.

On the other hand, a skilled psychiatrist who in a few hours of sessions on the couch has relieved a schizophrenic of the hallucination of voices may be a very reluctant recruit to the orthomolecular types of treatment. Those of you who know that there is a school of psychiatry which insists that we must view man holistically will wonder if these practitioners are not more likely to take the long perspective. They don't; in their philosophy, it is necessary to view both the effect of his environment on man, and the effect of man on his environment—but they do not ordinarily consider the *internal* environment. So, in this sense, the orthomolecular approach is simply an effort to take into consideration, as a possible cause of man's psychiatric troubles, one aspect of his environment which has received unhealthful neglect: THE INFLUENCE OF BODY ON MIND.

It is more than passing strange to say that we need to be reminded that the body influences the mind. Yet, a quick review of the introduction of the concept of the psychosomatic—the influence of mind on body—will give the reader a useful perspective. It was in the 1920s that Dr. Smith Ely Jeliffe, before the New York Academy of Medicine, proposed the concept that emotional and mental disturbances can create physical illness. His professional listeners suggested mockingly that he join the Christian Science Church, and his widow, with whom I have corresponded, tells me that he died with a broken heart. From mocking this new idea, which we now call psychosomatic medicine, the profession in adopting it swung completely to the other extreme, and the diagnosis of something "psychosomatic" very often became a monument to the physician's inadequacy as a diagnostician.* In the words of one observer, at the height of this movement you had to crawl into the physician's office on hands and knees to persuade him that whatever was wrong with you was not "all in your mind." As resistant as the profession was to the idea that mind has an influence on body, so tenacious is it, as the pendulum now swings in the other direction, in refusing to examine the corollary of the equation: disturbances of the body and its chemistry can warp thinking and distort emotions and derange perceptions—which is what this book is all about. One may anticipate that fifty years from now, an author will be struggling to remind the professions that mind also has an influence on body.

For those who cling to the concept that diseases of the mind owe nothing to disorders of the body, we should spend a few minutes with the evidence which clearly indicts derangement of body chemistry as a cause of psychosis. At the height of pellagra, a disease known to derive from dietary deficiency, the sufferer is plainly psychotic, and returns to sanity only when the dietary deficiencies have been rectified. Even before outright pellagra appears—while the patient shows no *physical* sign of the impending toll of inadequate diet—he complains of feeling "swimmy-headed," and, five years or more before a competent diagnosis of pellagra can be made, he is complaining that he hears voices which are not there. Some of his symptoms so closely resemble those of schizophrenia that they served as an inspiration for the use

---

*This is tragically illustrated in the history of a group of more than one hundred patients whose complaints had been dismissed as "psychosomatic," more than twenty-five of whom subsequently died of cancer. Examination of every one of the other patients revealed the presence of physical diseases which were responsible for the "psychosomatic" symptoms.

of the anti-pellagra vitamins in the therapies which became orthomolecular psychiatry.

In the blood of a large percentage of schizophrenics there appears a foreign chemical, originally called "the mauve [pink] spot." Injections of this factor into the blood stream of normal individuals—in one case, a psychiatrist—were followed by symptoms of schizophrenia. Fascinatingly, injections of the blood of human schizophrenics into spiders cause them to spin an abnormal and asymmetrical web, inevitably reminiscent of the distortions which are seen in the art work of human schizophrenics.

Studies of the incidence of schizophrenia in families show a predisposition to the disorder when it is present in the family history. This was, inevitably, initially attributed to environment, though common sense would indicate that environment does not descend unaltered through generation after generation.

Dr. Linus Pauling has shown that schizophrenics often demonstrate an abnormal need for the vitamins which have been found helpful in treating the disorder. He has, in fact, developed a test in children which may roughly indicate the probability that the disease will develop. It is predicated on the percentages of large doses of these vitamins which are retained by the child. The tendency to retain rather than to excrete very large doses of certain vitamins is related to increased likelihood of the development of schizophrenia.

It is exciting to realize that the proper choice of foods and vitamin-mineral supplements may return a neurotic to full function or a psychotic to the world of reality, and still more exciting to realize that there is great promise here for mentally retarded, autistic, withdrawn, and hyperactive children. It seems to me, though, that the most glowing of the possibilities offered by orthomolecular medicine and psychiatry is their application to improvement of the *normal*. Even the sophisticated layman with an all consuming interest in this research seems unaware of the rewards it offers in helping people who are *not* ill toward achievement of potentials they do not even know they possess—a process which is described in this book. Approach it without prejudice. You might remember that the Japanese, before World War II, thought that their small stature was dictated by their genes. With the introduction of improved nutrition, Japanese children, growing taller than their parents, clearly demonstrated that the ceiling was set by the national diet rather than Japanese chromosomes. Question: how do *you* know to what extent and in what subtle ways *you* are falling short of *your* potential because you have been persuaded that corn flakes, butylhydroxytoluene (BHT), hamburgers, milk shakes, and cola drinks provide the ideal internal environment?

I must emphasize here the observation made by many orthomolecular physicians and nutritionists who have seen improvement in *normal* patients, non-hypoglycemics, who have adopted the diet for low blood sugar. This may be interception of the beginning of the processes leading to hypoglycemia; it may reflect improvement of liver function, or relief of the adrenal glands from their long struggle with the overload of processed starches and sugars common in the American diet; it may spring from reduction of the intake of dubious food additives; it might be, very simply, the response to improved nutrition, but it is a real and satisfying gain which should remind us that we tend to confuse the *average* with the *normal.* I often think, in this context, of two patients in a sanitarium for which I was clinical nutritionist, to whom we gave supplementary amounts of niacinamide and Vitamin B complex. Though they exhibited none of the "classical" symptoms of deficiency in the vitamins, both patients reported that for the first time in their lives, they didn't feel "swimmy-headed," but were thinking clearly. When they left the institution, both patients subsequently were told by physicians to discontinue the supplements. After all, said the doctors, neither had pellagra.

When the head lama in *Lost Horizon* was asked why he permitted other churches to operate in a Shangri-la owned by his order, he replied that he moderately believed there is a moderate amount of truth in all pathways to the truth. Fortunately for many troubled children, one of the psychiatrists with that philosophy paused to take a long and critical look at the correspondence reaching him from hundreds of mothers of autistic, disturbed, and hyperactive children. In explaining why he had become an orthomolecular pediatric psychiatrist, he said that over a period of years, entirely independent of each other, many mothers began to give their aberrant children supplements of vitamins. The psychiatrist noted two other tendencies: the women tended to gravitate toward the same vitamins, and they reported that their children were substantially helped. Fascinatingly, the vitamins toward the use of which these mothers gravitated were largely those which Hoffer, Osmond, and other pioneers in orthomolecular psychiatry were prescribing in schizophrenia and other psychoses.

At a recent medical convention, I had the honor of being chairman of a panel in which orthomolecular therapy was discussed by a group of distinguished psychiatrists. As I left the platform, a St. Louis physician intercepted me, and said: "When you write a book on this subject, please emphasize the usefulness of this approach for patients who are not psychotic, not neurotic, but *are* nervous and having difficulty in coping with everyday stresses. I used to write," he said "over one thousand prescriptions a month for tranquilizers. It's down to fifty now." Just by way of letting you know that the battle is far from over, let me quote an administrative bulletin which was distributed to psychiatrists in a public institution, who were beginning to explore the usefulness of dietary control and megavitamin prescriptions for their psychotic patients. The bulletin in essence said: If you wish to prescribe any of the psychoenergizers, antidepressants, or tranquilizers (all capable, the bulletin did not remind the physicians, of causing serious and irreversible damage to brain and nervous systems) you are entirely free to do so. If you wish to prescribe vitamins and hypoglycemia diets, you are engaged in experimental medicine, and must obtain informed consent from the patients. When this was reported to me, I thought of the wards filled with patients with tardive dyskinesia, a deplorable side-reaction to psychotropic drugs—so common an effect that it is routinely listed as a warning to the physician in all advertising of psychotropic drugs—and suggested that perhaps the administration in the institution needed orthomolecular therapy more than the patients.

Make no mistake: this book presents no panacea. It does offer a new level of hope from a new kind of help.

·2·

When Allergy Assaults Sanity

FOR MORE THAN SIX YEARS, a New York City pharmacist, Irving Willner, has been filling orthomolecular vitamin prescriptions. He has little patience with physicians and psychiatrists who discount this new approach to mental disease.

"They ought to stand behind my counter for a few months," he suggested. "They'd change their minds. When the prescriptions for megadoses of vitamins first started to come in, I kept an open mind—I just watched what happened. The patients at first came in with friends or relatives, who waited for the prescriptions to be filled. I had to learn to be patient with emotionally disturbed kids, and not to get upset with the withdrawn ones whose minds seemed to be turned off, or in another world. The older ones either talked continuously, or they didn't respond at all when I tried to communicate with them. Some of them, of course, acted and talked normal, but some couldn't stand still—they wandered around the store. Sometimes their eyes looked unfocussed, or were too bright, or glassy, as if the kids were on hard drugs—which, I suppose, some of them might have been. Usually, most of them were dirty, with their hair wild, and some looked as if they hadn't bathed in months. For the first few refills, the parent or the friend would come back alone, and then the patients began to drift in, by themselves. They were cleaned up or cleaning up, and talking cheerfully, and telling me their stories. There were too many to remember, but there's one kid, a teenage girl, I'll never forget. She'd been severely schizophrenic, and had a history of three or four attempts at suicide, and she'd been violent. She called me long-distance—from Mexico City, I think it was—and said there was nothing wrong—just that I was the only person, other than her psychiatrist, who knew her history, and she just had to tell me—or someone—how good it feels to feel good.''

Willner's prescription files, by the accident of his store being near the offices of several pioneering orthomolecular psychiatrists, were among the first to reflect this revolution in psychiatric treatment. Practitioners whose prescriptions had listed tranquilizers, antidepressants, psychic energizers, and sleeping pills were now writing for heroic doses of vitamins—particularly niacin, niacinamide, Vitamin B_6, and Vitamins C and E, sometimes accompanied by concentrates of protein and supplements of trace minerals.

However, as research progressed, the practitioners became increasingly aware that cerebral allergy plays a dominant part in a large percentage of mental and emotional disorders; that it may not only cause neurotic and psychotic symptoms, but also may induce low blood sugar and nutritional deficiencies, which in turn reinforce the abnormal symptoms. Then the prescriptions began to mirror the highly individual sensitivities of patients who had proved allergic to the ordinarily innocuous fillers and binders used in all vitamin pills and capsules. The pharmacist had to meet these special needs through his own resources—there were no commercial ones, at that time—by creating nutritional concentrates free of corn starch, lactose, and other conventional fillers. "When they respond," Willner said thoughtfully, "it's worth all the effort. And a lot of them get better."

Most people know that allergy can cause symptoms like hay fever, asthma, hives, and some colds. But how is depression initiated or aggravated by the corn starch used as an "inert" filler in a vitamin pill? Why would milk sugar, normal to milk, and another of the "inert" ingredients in some pills and tablets, help to drive a patient deeper into delusions of persecution? This chapter gives some of the answers, tracing the connection between food additives and hyperactivity, between food intolerance and madness.

It is strange that the mass insanity which is modern warfare was responsible for a new understanding of one of the forces making for schizophrenia. Yet so it was, for during World War II, marked improvement occurred in Greek schizophrenics and paranoids when bread, a staple of the Greek diet, became scarce during the Nazi occupation.

It long had been known that the protein of bread (gluten) or one of its fractions cannot be tolerated by patients with celiac disease, and that celiacs tend to react to bread with both physical *and* psychological disturbances. Observers reported that the emotional symptoms of celiacs are usually the first to improve on a gluten-free diet. The stage was therefore set for instant recognition of the way in which the wartime shortage of bread had benefited Greek schizophrenics. One investigator has even speculated on the possibility that the aberrant genes that convey celiac disease may include one or more associated with schizophrenia. For there is overwhelming evidence that the tendency to schizophrenia *is* heritable—identical twins, for instance, tend to share it; fraternal twins may not.

The clue offered by the observations in Greece was followed by a psychiatrist who deleted wheat from the diets of hospitalized schizophrenics, and was able to prove that this one simple step had reduced the average period of hospitalization by a significant degree. Yet, by way of demonstrating the infuriating cultural lag created by the almost automatic resistance to new ideas in psychiatry, medicine, and nutrition, bread remains a staple of the diet in our overcrowded institutions, while administration of tranquilizers—which inflict irreparable harm on 12 percent of the schizophrenics who are dosed with them on a long-term basis—continues.

The appreciation of physical entities that make for mental dysfunction was heightened by another chance observation. Most of us have heard of babies born with an enzyme deficiency impairing their ability to metabolize phenylalanine, one of the essential amino (protein) acids conveyed by most animal proteins, with mental retardation as the penalty. But this discovery led to another: there are adults of normal intelligence who share this difficulty in the body's chemical "handling" of the amino acid. For them, the penalty is sporadic outbursts of major psychotic illness. Such research hopefully will spare these patients unnecessary electric convulsive treatments, tranquilizers, and psychiatric therapies.

The realization that allergy to foods and environmental factors may be the root of neurotic and psychotic behavior was likewise but recently born. It was the product of medical serendipity—the chance observation that had meaning to the prepared mind. There was a psychiatrist who counted himself as especially skillful in helping patients with fears and anxieties they could not justify or understand. He found that many of them could be trained out of their phobias by the standard technique of relaxation while approaching the terrifying situations through imagery. One of his successes was a woman with many irrational fears and a strong death wish, but the victory was temporary, for she reappeared at his office with all her phobias back, her wish to die overwhelming, and her eyelids so swollen that she could barely see. The referring physician, whom she had consulted because of her bloated eyelids, indicated that she was suffering from hypoglycemia (low blood sugar) because of overproduction of insulin.*

The psychiatrist assumed that this complication was psychosomatic, and "would vanish under my expert psychotherapy." He tested her for hypoglycemia, and found that her blood glucose (sugar) had dropped to half of what it should have been, at which point her depression and suicidal drive intensified. (He subsequently learned, in testing 600 psychiatric patients for hypoglycemia, that even mild drops in blood

---

*In Chapter Six, you will find a brief explanation of hypoglycemia (low blood sugar) and in Part II, Chapter One, a more detailed description of the condition and the tests used to diagnose it. It is *not* caused by lack of sugar in the diet.

sugar produced many of the symptoms of which the patients complained. But low blood sugar, he was to discover, is but one factor in the complicated relationship between body and mind.)

The swollen eyelids proved an important clue, though its meaning was not pieced together until after seven years of investigation. The swelling was based on food allergy, and the psychiatrist was astonished to realize that the allergic reaction involved not only the eyelids, but the brain itself. Moreover, that reaction caused the low blood sugar, and the two—hypoglycemia and allergic reactions in the brain—then combined to create the patient's fears, anxieties, and depression.

It has long been known that hypoglycemia may initiate or worsen allergy, though the implication of the discovery certainly has not been acted upon by allergists. Now we see that allergy may initiate hypoglycemia. As allergy can cause swelling of the skin (hives) so can it cause swelling of the brain, for which there is little tolerance in the rigid confines of the skull. (Such allergic swelling of the brain has been observed during surgery on susceptible individuals.) The pressure, of course, can cause symptoms. But allergy also involves profound impacts upon the chemistry of the body, the nervous system, and the brain—as any one knows who has experienced irritability after eating an offending food. In those who are so predisposed, the penalty for this reaction may be the initiation or aggravation of neurotic, paranoid, and/or schizophrenic behavior. None of these statements will carry the dramatic impact of watching the process at work—seeing a quiet, normal patient turned into a depressed, suicidal, or violent psychotic after a test done (under the tongue) of a food to which he is allergic—and the equal impact of reversal of the entire process by intravenous injections of Vitamin C and Vitamin B_6.

In years of study of the patient, the psychiatrist came to realize that when the troublemaking foods are withdrawn from or properly spaced in the diet, multiple symptoms of allergy, hypoglycemia, and addiction usually fade, as well as those attributed to nutritional deficiency and to inborn errors of metabolism (such as the mishandling of phenylalanine, referred to previously). The term ''addiction'' in this context does not refer to drugs, necessarily. It is used because, apparently paradoxically, patients with food allergies are often addicted to and eat large quantities of the very foods which are causing or aggravating their troubles. This comes about because the early reaction to an allergenic food may be a marked stimulation, of which the patient may be aware only on a subconscious level. One sign of the stimulation may be acceleration of the pulse, which is the rationale for the pulse-rate test for allergy. The patient, addicted to the food because of the lift it gives him, even if he is not consciously aware of the process, likewise does not realize that the price for the stimulation later may be fatigue, nervousness, irritability, fears, rage, or the full panoply of perceptual distortions of time, sound, space, and reality which are characteristic of schizophrenia.

These depressed, suicidal, fearful, and schizophrenic people whose troubles arise from allergy coupled with hypoglycemia are not a small minority. This mechanism is operating in at least 40 percent of all schizophrenics, and the actual figure may be as high as 60 percent. Rather than regarding this as a startling discovery, we should be willing to acknowledge that recognition of the role of allergy in behavioral problems is long overdue. Over twenty years ago, I observed in scanning the medical records of children in a home for ''juvenile delinquents'' that more than 60 percent of them had numerous and severe allergies, an incidence higher than one would anticipate in a similar group of average children. It never occurred to me, at the time, that some of their ''asocial behavior'' was in fact based on their allergies. I had a second opportunity to arrive at that conclusion when allergists, reporting in a symposium in Europe, demonstrated that they could turn asocial behavior on and off in children, by feeding or withholding foods to which they were allergic. Hindsight remains, as always, twenty-twenty.

Studies of hundreds of patients with neurotic or psychotic

behavior have now been made by allergists and psychiatrists, covering many diagnostic categories, and clearly indicating that a large percentage of troubled adults and children owe some—and not infrequently, a large majority—of their symptoms to allergy. An authority in the field found 92 percent of the schizophrenics to show evidence of cerebral allergy, producing major symptoms. The most frequent of the offending foods were the grasses—wheat, rye, oats, and barley—and the most common symptom was delusions of persecution, which strict Freudians commonly blame on latent or overt homosexuality. A study of children with behavioral or learning problems showed 80 percent to be allergic to corn. When these children, who were largely non-schizophrenic, were challenged with (tested with a dose of) corn, specific symptoms relating to their problems were sometimes produced. Children with dyslexia (problems in reading) were similarly affected. The same has been found true of hyperactive children, who prove routinely allergic, usually to one or more of the cereal grains, or milk, or both. There is evidence, too, that the child may react not only to the foods, but frequently to the additives accompanying them in processed foods, and to the insecticide residues with which they legally may be contaminated. Psychotic behavior has been the result of exposure to a *single* insecticide, in susceptible individuals. The reaction to additives may be pharmacological—a drug effect, a symptom of toxicity—rather than allergy. Selection of foods without additives is complex, and for that reason I have devoted the latter part of this chapter to guidance in the selection of such foods, on the urging of the many correspondents in the general public, the professions, and institutional staffs whose queries spurred the writing of this book.

The overlapping of low blood sugar with allergy in causing symptoms of neurosis and psychosis is striking. Disturbances accurately attributed to hypoglycemia could also be evoked in the same patients by specific foods—moreover, sometimes without a change in the level of blood sugar. I have already pointed out that hypoglycemia may cause or worsen allergy, as allergy may initiate or worsen hypoglycemia. There is a logical corollary: low blood sugar may disappear when the foods to which the patient is allergic and addicted are withdrawn from his diet. In fact, some of the recoveries we have attributed to the hypoglycemia diet may actually have accrued from its restrictions. Hypoglycemics are always forbidden to use sugar, and are urged to avoid caffeine, tobacco, junk foods, foods with additives and pesticide residues, etc. This is to say that in some cases, the therapeutic effect of the diet for low blood sugar came from cessation of the intake of foods to which the patient was allergic, though the dispensing physician or psychiatrist may not have been aware of the modality. On the other hand, some patients who have not fared well in treating hypoglycemia with the conventional high protein diet may be sensitive to certain amino (protein) acids; then the protein foods usually (and properly) emphasized in the dietary control of low blood sugar may aggravate it and the symptoms blamed on it. It must be remembered, also, that hypoglycemia—of itself, and in the absence of allergy—can cause highly neurotic or psychotic behavior, including unprovoked anxiety, suicidal depression, claustrophobia, insomnia, difficulty in concentrating, nervousness, fatigability, irritability, impotence, and frigidity—among some seventy symptoms reported by medical nutritionists and psychiatrists specializing in the diagnosis and treatment of low blood sugar.

The petroleum shortage which catalyzed the energy crisis may be a blessing to some of the depressed, neurotic, and psychotic, for petrochemicals—hydrocarbons derived from oil—are frequent offenders in initiating such symptoms. After deliberate exposure to automobile exhaust, one patient was suddenly persuaded that he was Jesus—a symptom easily "explained" by analysts as compensation for deep-seated feelings of great inferiority; another searched frantically to find a way to kill herself. An orthomolecular psychiatrist (who previously treated his patients with conversation-on-the-couch) shows a film of this girl, in which initially she appears perfectly normal, both in psychiatric testing and in everyday behavior. Merely inhaling the vapor from the ink in a marker pen—a petrochemical—caused loss of control of her speech, and rolling of her eyes, and impairment, despite her best efforts, of both gross and fine motor control. Vitamin C, used successfully as a detoxifying agent for these chemically defective patients, brought no response, but when Vitamin B_6 was added, results were immediate. Many orthomolecular psychiatrists have had this result with these two vitamins, given intravenously and by mouth. Other helpful procedures have been developed: the use of carbon dioxide and oxygen, or a balancing (weak) dose of the offending substance. The important point is this: the orthomolecular psychiatrist and the neurological allergist can literally turn on and off behavior which their peers are trying to interpret as "interpersonal conflict," treat with antidepressants and tranquilizers, or stamp out with shock therapy.

Understandably, practitioners who have diagnosed and successfully treated hundreds of hypoglycemic and allergic people on these bases believe that the marriage of biochemistry and behaviorism has placed psychiatry in a new and exciting era. One practitioner, deep in long-term productive research in the relationship of allergy and hypoglycemia to the problems of the schizophrenic, depressed, manic, withdrawn, neurotic, and hyperactive, has flatly stated that the majority of the emotionally disturbed are also chemically disturbed, and that correction of the physical disturbance is therapeutic for the mental and emotional. What he finds—and, I'm sure, you and I find—exciting is something less than that for his peers in the establishment. In a later chapter you will learn exactly how orthodox psychiatry is resisting acceptance of this breakthrough, and actually attempting to obstruct the research. Why are you, a psychiatrist, practicing allergy? What right have you to administer a fast? They sound as if psychiatry and psychoanalysis were craft unions, determined to prove the superiority of their particular techniques, however demonstrably ineffective.

In our highly chemicalized environment, there are literally millions of substances to which we are exposed daily. Consider some 3,000 additives in our foods, with new ones marketed every day. Consider the implications of the discovery that the residue from repeatedly distilled Boston drinking water proved mutagenic for seedlings. The body having had no physiological experience with these chemical invaders, it is not particularly astonishing that the sensitive and the chemically defective organism may react to one or a hundred of them; nor that the target organ in some of these people may be the brain; nor that the process may sometimes produce symptoms inviting the straitjacket or the shock table. Take a familiar odor: that of a new car. That aroma reflects the presence of at least fifty chemicals, many of them petroleum-based, to which some people react with physical distress or serious disturbances of the nervous system and brain. There are dozens of insecticides, many of them petrochemicals and many petroleum-borne, which cling to our fruits and vegetables, any one of which is capable of causing serious reactions in sensitive individuals. As one text on allergy remarks, over and over again: nothing is safe for everyone—a proposition which deserves more consideration from fluoridationists, marketers of additive-laden foods, and the government agencies devoted to their causes. The reactivity of highly allergic people passes belief. Theron Randolph, M.D., who was a pioneer in neuroallergy (and struggled for years to capture the attention of his peers), tells the story of a woman who, without leaving her bedroom on the second floor of her home, had a severe allergic reaction to a fungicide residue on oranges which were in a *closed* paper bag, in a first-floor kitchen. The response to the chlorine in drinking water can be depression or diarrhea, or both. The journals of allergy record reactions to the small amount of fluoride used in city water, though proponents of fluoridation insist that no one can react adversely to this very active chemical. While penicillin allergy is as familiar to the public as to the professions, and allergy to molds is a routine finding in tests, it is little appreciated by layman or psychiatrist that reaction to a fungus may take the shape of an emotional or mental disorder.

Years ago, as a token of our understandable ignorance (it is our pretensions which are unforgivable), we placed brain-injured children who were mentally normal in the same class-rooms with the retarded, though their problems in learning are a scholastic world apart. We are now making parallel errors in other types of learning difficulties. A psychiatrist tells the story of a young woman who had difficulties in learn-ing which could have easily been mistaken for a schizo-phrenic distortion of reality. When she tried to read, she complained that the words moved around the page, making it difficult for her to concentrate. When tested with a com-bination of corn and milk, she was then totally unable to read because, as she described it, a few words would fill an entire page. Petroleum hydrocarbons, alcohol, and the fumes of au-tomobile exhausts aggravated this problem, and brought on weakness and unsteadiness. Her hobby was painting, but a few pleasurable hours of that activity caused excessive per-spiration, loss of strength, and a rash, the reaction lasting several days. She remained symptom-free only when wet paint was completely removed from her environment.

Aware that such reactions must seem startling to the lay-man, let me point out that they should not be to allergists. Their journals have long recorded equally violent reactions in other systems of the body. I am thinking of the case re-ported, long ago, in which a physician at intervals totally lost his hearing in both ears. The mischief-maker turned out to be tomato juice, of which he was fond. One four-ounce glass was enough; thirty minutes later the patient was totally deaf, the effect lasting for a number of hours.

A striking example of a family where allergy to the same foods caused widely different symptoms in different individ-uals, ranging from the purely physical to the purely mental or emotional, is found in a psychiatrist's history of a woman who developed ulcerative colitis, followed by psychotic symptoms. Her problems were traced to an intolerance for wheat. Her fourteen-year-old son's paranoid behavior disap-peared likewise when wheat was removed from his diet. Her ten-year-old, whose hallucinations led him to believe the clouds in the sky were talking to him, also owed his delusions to wheat intolerance, and when the grain was removed from his menus, his hyperactivity, behavior problems, and poor learning also disappeared. For such people "a little wheat" is like "a little carbolic acid," but avoiding it isn't easy. Bread is an obvious source, and so are cereals, but how many processed foods contain wheat flour or wheat starch, unannounced on the label because there is a "Standard of Identity" resting in the F.D.A. files in Washington?

Another woman had undergone lengthy and unhelpful psychiatric treatment for "neurosis" based on "interpersonal conflict." A loading test in which she took 9,000 mgs. of Vitamin C in twenty-four hours indicated that her body had retained and used 7,560 mgs., excreting the small remainder. Such retention, frequent in schizophrenia, is far beyond the amount retained by normal individuals. Significantly, when toxic agents and allergenic substances are removed from the diet and environment, the percentage of retained Vitamin C will drop steadily, as an indication that the body is returning to normal.

The patient strongly resisted the concept that her many "emotional" troubles were in any way and any part based on allergy. The psychiatrist commented that this was an attitude certainly removing the possibility of the power of suggestion as determining her numerous adverse reactions to common foods. Corn gave her nasal clogging, a postnasal drip, sleepiness, coughing, and depression. After drinking milk, she burped, passed gas, complained that her head felt weird, her ears became plugged, and she developed an uncontrollable diarrhea. With wheat, the nasal symptoms of corn allergy were repeated, her voice became hoarse, her cheeks flushed, and her tongue sore. She was highly allergic to the grass family—wheat, rye, oats, and rice. Tests for these and other foods caused marked restlessness, a speech difficulty which made it hard for her to express herself, depression, shortening of her concentration span, and inability to think clearly. Neither her psychiatric treatment nor therapy for her hypoglycemia had benefited her, and even those professional men stubbornly resistant to the concept that the body influences the mind will acknowledge that removal of these disturbing foods from the patient's internal environment must help her in responding to the conventional psychiatric therapy she may also need.*

For a few years Russian psychiatrists have been reporting successful use of prolonged fasts in the treatment of schizophrenia. They observed significant reduction in the number and intensity of psychotic symptoms in patients maintained only on water for thirty days, though they acknowledged that return to a normal diet tended to cause the disturbances to reappear. On that basis, they amended their procedure by suggesting that such patients should return to a "prophylactic" fast for four or five days, once a month. Some American orthomolecular psychiatrists promptly adopted the technique, with the same initial successes and the same reappearance of symptoms when the fasts were broken. I took a dim view of the concept, for schizophrenics are notoriously ill-gaited for stress, and fasting is indubitably a pronounced one—until I realized that the fast removed from the patients' internal environments *all* foods and beverages, all additives and insecticide residues to which they were allergic. This in turn explained the renascence of the symptoms when normal diet was restored. A similar procedure in the treatment of multiple, intractable allergies was used by American allergists for many years. It began with a sparse diet, limited to foods to which allergies are rare. New foods were added, one at a time, with sufficient intervals to allow the physician to appraise accurately the response to each. The Russians had not, then, discovered an arcane effect of fasting on psychosis. Their error lay in restoration of a full diet shortly after the termination of the fast. Had they added foods singly, with sufficient spacing, they might have realized that the responses

---

*Lest you think that resistance to innovation in psychiatric therapies is a phenomenon confined to the old guard in that discipline, consider the warning Natalie Golos, author of *Management of Complex Allergies*, thought necessary to give her readers, individuals tortured with neuroallergy simulating every mental and physical disease: "If you find your doctor derisive . . ."

of their fasting patients reflected relief from symptoms of allergy.

The fasting technique is useful, then, when patients are severely allergic to an overwhelming number of foods. This is illustrated in the history of a young woman who had been suicidal and homicidal for years, attempting to kill herself and her parents, always depressed, and sometimes catatonic. Electric convulsive and megavitamin therapies yielded no improvement, nor did five hospitalizations and psychiatric treatment by three psychiatrists, successively. She was then tested for vitamin deficiencies and biochemical disturbances. Deficiency in niacin was confirmed; excretion of galactose, a form of sugar, was twelve times normal; a Vitamin C loading test showed that she retained more than 7,500 mgs. of a 9,000-mg. dose (in twenty-four hours), revealing that the body needed detoxification. In tests for specific allergies, she developed a constellation of symptoms. Exposure to a common insecticide caused tenseness, nervousness, and depression. Exposure to chlorine in the concentration usual to city drinking water depressed her to the point of saying, over and over again: "I want to die!" Her hands at that time broke out in perspiration, she felt cold, and she complained of difficulty in breathing. Many such symptoms were produced by saccharin, automobile exhaust, banana, lamb, watermelon and other fruits, and molds. Her sensitivity to petrochemicals was so exquisite that it negated benefit from megavitamin therapy, since the vitamin formulations, her psychiatrist noted, sometimes contain such compounds. This girl, he observed, is chemically a defective person—which might be translated as deficiency in some of the enzyme systems which help you and me to survive in a contaminated world. But with special care and precautions, the girl is now in college, a normal and outgoing person, with no evidence of catatonia, feelings of inferiority, or attacks of depression. Her doctor regards her allergies and toxic reactions to environmental factors as good illustrations of what a psychiatrist doesn't know about his patients. Which is forgivable—if the psychiatrist does not, out of hand, reject these concepts without examining them.

When hypoglycemia is present and unrecognized, which is also unpardonable when the test is readily available and the remedies at hand, the patient may likewise spend fruitless years in costly psychiatric therapy. Such was the experience of a member of the faculty of a major university, who wrote to tell me of his frustrating experience with an "anxiety neurosis" which, accompanied by great irritability and fatigability, threatened to incapacitate him completely. Three years of psychoanalysis made the analyst feel much better, but the professor's condition had not improved under the therapeutic impact of questions like: "And what incident in your childhood did this remind you of?" Then the educator happened on my book on hypoglycemia. Though as a professor of English he wasn't likely to be overwhelmed by *any* book, as he remarked in his letters to me, he was startled by the many ways in which the text seemed to be describing him. He asked his physician to give him the test for hypoglycemia, for which the doctor referred him to a large hospital, a teaching institution associated with a medical school. The graph of his blood levels of sugar, after a large dose of it, not only showed a sharp *drop* in a short time, but the patient had serious reactions *during the test*—which is irrefutable evidence that the hypoglycemia is responsible for the symptoms. As his blood sugar descended with abnormal speed—a phenomenon more meaningful than the level at any given time—the professor went into convulsions, which were succeeded by stuttering, which was followed by his losing all color vision, and seeing everything in black and white. These symptoms were duly noted at the appropriate points on the chart of the glucose tolerance test, which the administering physician signed. Over his signature was this immortal comment: "Glucose tolerance normal"! I sent a copy of the graph and the comments to a medical nutritionist who specializes in hypoglycemia. He pronounced the test as confirming hypoglycemia, and the symptoms as indicating it to be a severe case. Of the comment by the physician who had signed the test, the specialist remarked, simply: "He is guilty of malpractice." I should be more inclined to place the responsibility on the medical and diabetes societies who have advised physicians that "hypoglycemia is a fad disease." They have created a climate in which these pioneers in neurological allergy, hypoglycemia, and orthomolecular psychiatry will face the most difficult of all educational challenges: that of teaching physicians who don't know, but think they do.

Recently, in an informal discussion at a meeting of the Academy of Orthomolecular Psychiatry, a Canadian pediatrician spoke of his experience with hyperactive children. For the first time in his practice, he had administered megadoses of vitamins for a hyperactive child, who was so disturbed that he was uncontrollable at home and ineducable in school. Constant doses of amphetamines kept him under precarious control. (Treatment with a stimulant to produce sedative effects rests upon the paradoxical chemistry of a child's nervous system, which, until it matures, reacts to sedatives with stimulation, to stimulants with sedative effects.) The mother was unhappy with the prospect of treating a child with a powerful stimulant over a period of years, but there was no escape—his behavior without medication was unbearable, and she surrendered, and sent him to school after a morning dose, and met him at the door, literally, on his return, with another.

The physician was willing to try high doses of niacin, Vitamin B_6, Vitamin E and Vitamin C, on the basis of the responses reported in Dr. Allan Cott's papers on the response of hyperactive, autistic, and withdrawn children to this harmless therapy, but he advised that the amphetamine be continued, along with the new vitamin treatment, for the first few weeks. In the initial four days of the combined therapy, the child showed a remarkable improvement, and then, literally, overnight, worsened so dramatically that his despairing mother asked the doctor for permission to stop the vitamins. "What intuition led me to stop the amphetamine, instead, I'll never know," he confessed. "I told her to drop the morning dose of the drug, and if that worked all right, to delay the homecoming dose by an hour more, each day. Well! He did just fine, and the delaying of the afternoon amphetamine pill by an hour each day gradually brought him up to bedtime without a dose, and then, of course, we could eliminate it entirely.'' He added, for the benefit of several laymen in the group: ''You see, the vitamin treatment had reversed the paradoxical response to the stimulant. It was now acting as a stimulant, and driving the child up a wall!'' He beamed with satisfaction, as might any pediatrician who succeeds in relieving a child of a potent dosage of a dangerous drug by the use of harmless vitamins.

Actually, the use of stimulant drugs for a hyperactive child is undesirable from any point of view. It is symptomatic treatment, which is never ideal, and the less so when the drug is possibly harmful. The child grows up with a drug personality, and his parents, peers, and teachers may never know him—and he may not know himself—as he really is. Most regrettable is the fact that the symptomatic treatment may be covering the real causes. His actual condition may be hypoglycemia, or he may have elevated lead levels in his blood, which, lead being a neurological poison, may worsen, if it doesn't actually cause, his hyperactivity. He may be the victim of neurological allergy—many of these children undoubtedly are. I have seen a single glass of a cola drink touch off an attack of hyperactivity lasting two days. Dr. Harry Swartz watched three days of hyperactivity follow consumption of a doughnut. The child's nervous system may be the victim of a pharmacological reaction to food additives, or even a reaction to a chemical normal to food, when it is related to a drug to which the child is sensitive. For example, a child allergic to aspirin may react to related compounds occurring naturally in certain foods.

It must be obvious, from the complexities of the problems of the patients whose histories you have read, that the management of sensitivity, neurological allergy, intolerances, and hypoglycemia as entities in neurotic and psychotic behavior is a complex medical and nutritional problem. Despite its complexity, a large part of the treatment falls ultimately into the hands of the parent, relative, or, in some cases, the patient himself, for eternal dietary vigilance is the price of freedom from the psychiatric couch, the mental hygiene institution, and the unending prescriptions for psychotropic drugs which threaten long-term, irreversible side-effects. Securing competent medical help is an equal problem. Allergists with a background in neurological allergy are a small group. The number of orthomolecular psychiatrists is growing, but not as fast as the number of prescriptions for tranquilizers, psychic energizers, antidepressants, and sleeping pills written by medical men who have neither backgrounds nor interest in nutrition, neurological allergy, orthomolecular psychiatry, or hypoglycemia. (Though sugar was recognized, among all foods, as being the prime source of troubles for patients with low blood sugar, and this more than *fifty* years ago, I still currently meet and hear from patients who have been told to eat candy as medication for their hypoglycemia.) Even in those quarters where competent help should immediately be available, it often isn't. As an example, consider this paragraph from a letter written by an intelligent man who discovered—through this own reading—that he might escape the psychiatric couch if he could find a physician competent in administering and interpreting a glucose tolerance test, and in acting upon his findings:

"It is distressing to me that so many medical men could be so misinformed about the nature of an illness as terrifying and incapacitating as this illness has been to me, and I fervently hope you will continue in your efforts to convince the medical profession that the established 'norms' for blood sugar are erroneous. Again, my thanks for your book. I only wish the staff at [name deleted] Hospital would read and believe it." He names a major teaching hospital. How well will their graduates serve other victims of the missed diagnosis, who actually owe their symptoms to hypoglycemia, but are being assured that they are neurotic?

The obvious purpose of this book—to acquaint you with the philosophy of the "right molecule," and the reasoning and experiences dictating it—will be fulfilled if through its information you are better equipped to follow the guidance of the practitioner—and are given at least a head start in finding your way to such professional men. For this reason, you will find in the Appendix, among other information, names of professional and lay groups who maintain lists of ortho-molecular psychiatrists, neurological allergists, and medical nutritionists competent in the management of hypoglycemia, nutritional deficiencies, and those inborn derangements of metabolism for which we have remedies.

What causes hypoglycemia (low blood sugar), how the tests for the condition are conducted, and what nutritional safe-guards the patient requires are spelled out in detail in Part II of this book, for it is critically important that there be com-petent management of those aspects of the problem which involve the home and the family menus. I urge you not to dismiss arbitrarily the possibility that hypoglycemia may be part of the difficulties of the schizophrenic, the depressed, the mentally retarded, the dyslexic, the autistic, the hyper-active, the slow learner, and the ''neurotic.'' The vast amount of sugar consumed by the public presents a burden beyond the capacity of the body to endure indefinitely, in many in-dividuals. Allergy to sugar, though rare, does occur, and may contribute to low blood sugar. The processing of sugar in-volves exposure to hydrocarbons, to which, as you have al-ready learned, many individuals are sensitive, and may react. On pages 124–25 you will find a listing of the symptoms triggered by abuse of sugar in the diet, and on pages 147–49 you will find a chart of the sources from which we derive an intake of sugar which may mount to 20 percent of the total calorie intake, in many diets. In helping the troubled child or adult, therefore, we must pay as much attention to the intake of sugar as we do to the more than five pounds of food additives each of us consumes per year.

In attempting to bar food additives from the diet of the hyperactive or allergic or hypoglycemic individual, you will find the task so complex that you will wonder why the phy-sician doesn't desensitize the patient against these factors, as he would with ragweed pollen shots for hay fever. This is impossible—there are too many additives; the formulas of foods (and additives used) change too frequently, and new additives are introduced almost daily. Example: your baker may use shortening with BHT in one batch, and BHA in the next. Our intake of chemicals forced upon us as additions to our foods has now passed five pounds per year, and that doesn't include the pesticide residues brought to us on major crops. Vigilance is the only safeguard—that, and a well-informed consumer.

Reading food labels is particularly important when biochemical disturbances are behind neurotic, psychotic, or behavioral problems. A medical man with one of the Kaiser groups discovered that the additives play an important part in starting or perpetuating hyperactivity. The ubiquitousness of food additives will be apparent when you realize that the medicine prescribed by your pediatrician may contain a coal-tar dye. The very antihistamine you take to relieve symptoms of allergy may be tinted blue or red with a coal-tar dye capable of touching off reactions in the sensitive; so may the vitamin tablet. The additives in baked goods may be potent enough to start trouble. The moral for this is simple: bake at home, know your ingredients, and enjoy the opportunity to make it more nutritious and lower in sugar than the commercial equivalents. When you're cooking for a hypoglycemic, *The Low Blood Sugar Cookbook,* by Francyne Davis, published by Grosset and Dunlap, will be helpful. For better nutrition and fewer additives in your cooking and baking, let me immodestly recommend my own *Carlton Fredericks Cookbook for Good Nutrition*—same publisher.*

Breakfast cereals—the most dispensable of all foods—are almost uniformly laden with undesirable preservatives, including the BHT previously discussed, as well as coal-tar dyes. Avoid any where "artificial flavor" or "artificial color" are mentioned, as well as those which indicate the presence of "freshness preservers," under which may hide BHA and

---

*Baked and other recipes for schizophrenics and others with wheat intolerance can be a problem. If other grains are tolerated, such as rice, you will find useful recipes in *Gourmet Food on a Wheat-Free Diet*, by Marion N. Wood, published by Charles C. Thomas. Many of the recipes, please note, are entirely too high in sugar, and you must experiment with using less. It's mandatory in many of the problems we've discussed.

BHT. The health food stores carry brands of granola which are additive-free, and the supermarkets now stock "natural cereals" which are also free of added chemicals, but contain so much sugar—20 to 30 percent—that they should not be labeled natural, and are nutritionally undesirable for children who are well, or for the hyperactive or the hypoglycemic.

Spray residues are almost inevitable on popular fruits, and the amount is *not* as minute as most people think. It is true that the F.D.A. limits the residue of this toxic insecticide or that to five parts per million, or less. It's true that when two insecticides of the same chemical family are present, the combined amount is limited to five parts per million, or so. But if the grower exercises all his options in the use of *different* kinds of insecticides, not of the same chemical family, the five parts per million ceiling holds for *each*. One expert estimated that the total residue on an apple might climb to more than two hundred parts per million—and remember that we are discussing highly toxic substances which, in company, may interact—for less toxicity, hopefully; for more, quite possibly. At any rate, spray residues of insecticides occur on cherries, apples, pears, apricots, nectarines, peaches, plums, currants, olives, strawberries, raspberries, blueberries, cranberries, boysenberries, rhubarb, and the citrus fruits—grapefruit, oranges, lemons, as well as grapes. Antifungal agents capable of causing severe allergic reactions will be found residual on some fruit. Jams and jellies made from fruits which carry pesticide residues may be contaminated, which is to say that cooking does not remove all, nor do ordinary washing, cleaning, and other household measures. Moral: if you can afford it, and I don't see how you can't when the average American household finds money for smokes and liquor and candy, you can usually obtain supplies of fruits and vegetables that have not been sprayed, at your local health food store.

Among the vegetables likely to have undergone heavy spraying: cauliflower, head lettuce, broccoli, hothouse tomatoes, mushrooms (particularly heavily sprayed with F.D.A. permission for higher residues), cabbage, spinach, asparagus, celery, mustard greens, beet greens, chard, escarole, loose-leaf lettuce, and endive. Chinese cabbage and artichoke may be guilty, too. Most root vegetables acquire spray residues only indirectly, through contamination of the soil via spraying of the leaves. Off flavors in carrots, for instance, are not uncommon, as a price for excessive spraying of the carrot tops, the run-off reaching the soil. These insecticides are often oil-soluble, invade the food, and resist your peeling, washing, soaking, and cooking. Detergents labeled as insecticide removers have no virtues not shared by any cleaning material the housewife ordinarily uses for dishes.

Among meats, insecticides tend to concentrate in the fat of lamb, beef, pork, and fowl. Chicken stock will reflect that concentration, passing it on to other ingredients in recipes. While the animals and fowl are rarely sprayed directly, they may be subjected to drift of these poisons from adjacent crop areas reaching their grazing grounds. In the feed lots, the animals—save on the rare truly organic farms—will be consuming insecticide residues in the mash, silage, or whatever. Spraying of barns is common practice, and this, too, may reach the animals.

Careful removal of the fat, where the insecticides tend to concentrate, would be prudent in preparing lamb, beef, pork, and fowl. Fowl is no longer treated with synthetic female hormone (which is about to go back into use in the beef industry) but chickens *are* dosed with arsenate compounds, which tend to accumulate in the liver. The arsenate people, understandably, do not disapprove of this, but a sensitive person's physiology might. Organically raised beef, pork, and fowl are sometimes available, but be sure of your source. We are buying more organic food than is being produced, which does not reflect on the health food retailer—who is as honest as other retailers—but on the fact that every industry, among its suppliers, must cope with the fast-dollar operators; the integrity of organic producers of food sans chemicals is difficult to verify.

Sulfur is widely used by food processors, and is a fertile source of trouble for the allergic and for the hyperactive. In one chemical form or another, sulfur is used to slow down the browning of fruits and french-fried potatoes; to bleach dried fruit; to retard mold in such foods as apricots, peaches, nectarines. It is also used in commercially prepared foods made from fresh apples, peaches, or apricots; fruit marmalades; corn syrup, corn oil, and corn starch.

Artificial colors run riot in colored ice cream, gelatin desserts, sherbet, cake, candy, topping and filling for cakes and pies, frankfurters, bologna, margarine, cheese, butter, Irish potatoes, sweet potatoes, yams, and soft drinks. Fruit juices are innocent, but when you buy "fruit punch" or "fruit drink" you are purchasing much added sugar, water, corn syrup, and artificial color, which is usually coal-tar in origin. (In most states, such junk is taxed as a soft drink, not as a food—take notice!) I have already mentioned the use of coal-tar dyes in pills—even vitamin pills. Some of them also contain preservatives and artificial sweetener. Apropos of remedies: there are supplements of natural origin available in health food stores. These vitamin preparations usually omit artificial color and preservatives. I stress this because I have found BHA, BHT, coal-tar dye, and saccharin in chewable vitamins on sale in supermarkets and drug stores—a battery of unnecessary hazards for a normal child, a real threat to the sensitive and hyperactive.

The emphasis on additives should not distract your attention from natural ingredients of food which may disturb sensitive individuals. Allergy to aspirin is so common that painkillers not based on salicylic acid have won a considerable market; but few consumers realize that this chemical is a natural constituent of such foods as apricots, prunes, peaches, plums, raspberries, grapes, oranges, cucumbers, and tomatoes. Helpful guidance in avoiding such foods when they are disturbing to those allergic to aspirin, as well as aid in identifying other drugs and chemicals which are potential troublemakers for the sensitive, may be obtained from the Allergy Foundation of Lancaster County, Box 1424, Lancaster, Pennsylvania 17604.

The exposure of foods to gas, deliberately or inadvertently, is a common practice in the food industry, and often a problem for the allergic. Apples, pears, and bananas are frequently ripened with ethylene gas. Coffee may be roasted over an open gas flame, exposing the consumer to ingestion of combustion products. Honey, though as much a threat to hypoglycemics and diabetics as any form of sugar, is less likely than most foods to carry insecticide residues, for the good reason that the bees do not survive exposure to them. Honey, like sugar, is often filtered through charcoal or bone char, making unclarified honey, obtainable in health food stores, a better choice for those sensitive to hydrocarbons. The clarification is a gratuitous hazard for the sensitive, aimed at the cosmetic effect of making the honey "clear," but also removing much of the small content of natural nutrients. Maple syrup, no more desirable a form of sugar than any other, may legally contain two parts per million of methyl formaldehyde, another threat to the sensitive. Raw, brown, and turbinado sugar offer no better nutrition than white sugar, other than a small content of chromium better obtained from superior foods; they present the same hazards to the chemically sensitive, and in the case of raw sugar, embellish the problem with the possibility that it may not be clean.

Distinct problems arise with plastics, which are treated with agents to make them flexible. These plasticizers tend to migrate—you transfer ten parts per million to your food when you handle it with disposable plastic gloves. As much as 60 percent of a plastic wrap may consist of plasticizer, which could be picked up by the fat or the protein of the food wrapped in the plastic. These include home-wrapped foods, and the pre-wrapped vegetables and salad greens, and so on, in the stores. Cellophane wrap is innocent of these dangerous chemicals, but other manufacturers have refused to give me any information, on the grounds of "trade secrets." There is the possibility that the most popular type of plasticizer may be toxic for healthy human beings; for the allergic, sensitive, and hyperactive, they are an unnecessary hazard. Other than cellophane, aluminum foil would be a safe selection. The plastic containers are also a possible problem. Many of these distinctly smell of plasticizer, but the absence of the odor does not mean that you're safe; filing the plastic will sometimes release the aroma, and warn you.

The glycols used in drying foods are occasional troublemakers, particularly in whole-wheat crackers and prepared coconut. Allergenic waxes are applied to turnips, apples, citrus fruits, eggplants, cucumbers, and green peppers.

Is the game worth the (petrochemical) candle? Indeed, it is: the hyperactive child has been known to recover completely when relieved of this gratutitous burden of chemical insult. The neurotic and psychotic symptoms of the chemically defective who cannot live with these chemicals will also improve.*

Though it is an understandable human tendency to seek a magic pill that will overnight (or in a few weeks, at the outside) cure the patient, these problems of hypoglycemia, neurological allergy, hyperactivity, and related neurotic and psychotic symptoms will require the long-term help of a group of experts. The point must be made that you will not yet find a single medical man whose skills include all the expertise in all the fields the patient needs. At the present state of the art, an orthomolecular psychiatrist, a neurological allergist, a medical nutritionist, and perhaps an expert in behavioral psychology will be the team needed; though occasionally, you will encounter a single practitioner who is competent in all or most of these fields, and wise enough to disclaim expertise where he falls short. It is for needed help in guiding you and your physician to practitioners skilled in medical nutrition, orthomolecular psychiatry, and neuroallergy that Section II of this book lists unbiased sources from which you can obtain the names of consultants. In that section, you will also find detailed descriptions of many of the tests used in psycho-nutrition, that you may more intelligently cooperate with the consultant of your choice.

*In *Look Younger, Feel Healthier,* published by Grosset & Dunlap in paperback, you will find further guidance in avoiding food additives and in food selection for better nutrition, both in the supermarket and the health food store.

·3·

The Chemical Nature
of the Beast

THE AVERAGE READER has a concept of schizophrenia leaning toward the "split personality" image of a Dr. Jekyll and Mr. Hyde. Actually, the sickness invokes a very different kind of rift—between thought and emotion, between thought and action—a cleavage which is quite apart from the problems of multiple personalities. From what you have already read, you will have realized that schizophrenia is not a single disorder, nor one for which the patient's spouse, siblings, or parents are to be blamed—unless you wish to hold them personally responsible for the genetic predisposition. Rather, schizophrenia is a blanket title for a group of biochemical disturbances which cause a kaleidoscopic array of psychiatric and physical symptoms, with the chemical aberrations differing from one group of schizophrenics to another, the common denominator being twisting of thinking and distortion of emotion based on derangement of the chemistry of the brain. If stress and other environmental factors play a role, it is obvious that the insult must fall upon a prepared soil.

Schizophrenics generally share perceptual distortions. Their senses of taste, hearing, vision, and smell transmit to them "realities" which do not exist but which appear very real, for the perceptions which are distorted reach the brain via the normal pathways. (If your thoughts appeared to be voices reaching your ears in the normal way, why would you realize that they are, in fact, of internal origin?) They are turned inward, understandably preoccupied exclusively with their internal turmoil. They are panicky without justification, anxious without external cause, and in a state of constant fear—fear of people, fear of their brains "boiling," fear of surviving in the hell in which they are living, and desperately afraid of coping with new situations. Their fatigue is constant and crippling, their headaches and insomnia frequently severe. Many of them have delusions of persecution, a symptom which terrifies normal people but actually is less troublesome to treat than many of their other twists in thinking. Some of them have loss of appetite and pronounced weight loss. Nearly all have distorted emotional responses, from no response (flat) to hysteria. Changes in personality are universal. Stress is their most bitter enemy.

In the preceding chapter, you came to realize that allergy and low blood sugar may interact (in either direction) to cause symptoms of psychosis. In the chapter you are about to read, you will encounter some of the types of schizophrenia which have been traced to specific disturbances in body chemistry, based on deficiency in Vitamin B_6 and zinc (metabolically, not dietetically, for there may be adequate supplies of the factors in the blood) or inadequate tissue supplies of Vitamin B_{12} (again, with normal levels in the blood). You begin to understand why tests for blood levels of vitamins are not always revealing. What is there may not reach the tissues; what is there may be within "normal range" and yet not adequate for the person's needs.

You will read, too, what happened when mothers, unable to obtain cooperation from their skeptical physicians in administering orthomolecular treatment to their autistic or disturbed children, undertook it on their own. You will come to realize from some of the histories in this chapter that some of the aged thrown on the scrap heap of "senile dementia" (second childhood) could be rescued, with vitamin-filled hypodermics.

You should emerge from this chapter with the realization that a straw man has been created by the establishment in psychiatry as it bitterly resists the orthomolecular concept.

Though the accusation has been made, no one, however justifiably enthusiastic about this new approach to ancient mental problems, has suggested that the institutions could be emptied if we poured enough of this vitamin or that into their psychotic populations. The chemistries of thinking and emotion are delicately balanced. Inadequate production of this enzyme or that can distort it. Excessive enzyme activity likewise disturbs the exquisite sequence of chemical events housed in the brain. Adequate intake—which may mean astronomical supplies—of the building materials for enzymes which are underproduced may induce the body to manufacture more. The production of the "wrong molecules" responsible for at least two types of schizophrenia may be chemically blocked by harmless intake of the appropriate vitamins. This makes it doubly ironic that the professionals who close their minds to the orthomolecular concept are actually using it when they prescribe tranquilizers, psychoenergizers, and antidepressants. They, too, are prodding enzyme production; they, too, are in pursuit of the wrong molecules, for which they are *using* the wrong molecules, as demonstrated by the appalling list of side reactions to the potent drugs they employ. What is worse: these mindbending drugs are symptomatic treatment, the practice of medicine at its worst, creating a drug-dependent population which, under its artificially induced calm, is as sick as ever it was.

It is with a jaundiced eye that Jill reads the psychiatric papers and texts she used in her training as a psychological therapist, for she herself suffered the agony of schizophrenia, and found her way out with the help of an orthomolecular psychiatrist. She describes herself as always an erratic and unstable person, given to highs as unjustified as the lows that followed them. As a veteran of her own two years of psychotherapy, and as an experienced practitioner, she was thoroughly familiar with neurotic and psychotic behavior, but that didn't stop her from drifting imperceptibly into the discovery that the world had become gray, colorless, and without dimension.

This was followed by pervasive fatigue and continuous severe headaches, which she did not associate with schizophrenia, in which they are frequent. Her neck was so tense she couldn't bear to hold her head up, and the left side of her body developed a numbness which at times immobilized her. Though she had been a very articulate person, her speech became hesitant, and she found herself both stuttering and losing control of the content of what she was saying. Her thoughts ran together, without structure or form. Hallucinations developed, followed by attacks which seemed almost epileptic. She felt that she was freezing internally, although it was imperceptible to her husband and physicians. Nausea was frequent, seeming to be brought on by an odor which penetrated her body like a gas, through the skin and orifices. Her mouth was parched, her tongue swollen, her irritability so intense that it had its impact not only on her, but her family.

She attempted to continue her practice, but her interviews with her patients suffered; she felt that she was not communicating with them. Weekends were lost, and then Fridays and Mondays followed them into a gray limbo. The climax came when she found herself catatonic, as though behind a glass wall, seeing, hearing, perceiving, but unable to respond, and at last, horrifiedly aware that she was involved in a psychotic process. With this realization, she determined that she would find help or kill herself, rather than permit her family to bear the burden of her affliction. That was the moment when she widened her search of the literature, seeking something more promising than drugs, psychotherapy, and electric convulsive treatments—and happened upon the first papers she had encountered on orthomolecular psychiatry.

Under the care of a psychiatrist experienced in this field she was tested for low blood sugar (hypoglycemia) which was present, as it is in some 60 percent of all schizophrenics. While no one blames hypoglycemia for causing the psychosis, its devastating impact on both the thinking and emotional brains must intensify the symptoms, interfere with the schizophrenic's tenuous grasp on reality, and obstruct his communication with his psychiatrist. She was placed on the conventional hypoglycemia diet: as low in sugar as possible, with a limited amount of the starches; the protein and the fat reasonably high. Vitamin C was given because schizophrenia reflects a toxic condition for which the vitamin in large doses is a partial antidote. Vitamin E, because it quiets anxiety without making a vegetable of the patient, as the drugs often do, and because it is useful in the treatment of depression. Niacin and niacinamide, aimed directly at the disturbed brain chemistry which is the essence of the type of schizophrenia Jill suffered. Vitamin B_6, as a detoxifying agent and for its roles in cerebral metabolism. Actually, three types of treatment were combined in this approach. One, aimed at compensating for deficiency in the nutrients. The second, aimed at dependency on the nutrients—satisfying requirements so high they could not possibly be satisfied with any selection of foods. The third, the use of the nutrients to block the body's synthesis of the "wrong molecules."

In response, Jill emerged from her colorless shadow world, with a clear understanding of what would have happened had she not found a practitioner aware that the body influences the mind. Had she been exposed to a compassionate and capable therapist, she observes, she might have learned to live with and to control her symptoms. But removal of the symptoms and restoration of the ability to live a normal life were more than she had ever hoped to gain. From the fruits of her experience, she draws a psychologist's conclusion for the benefit of other therapists and their patients. She points out that the approach to dealing with the schizophrenic processes *must* encompass *both* physical and mental levels. She warns that without this dual approach, the practitioner is condemning the mentally sick person to a lifetime spent under the burden of what can be an overwhelming handicap, which reaches out beyond the individual and contaminates those who surround him. And she adds that psychiatrists and psychologists are obligated to realize the inadequacies of their knowledge, and thereby remain open to new ideas and concepts, lest they markedly lessen their effectiveness. Her fellow therapists can learn from her.

Happily, the disturbed chemistries that make for psychosis are sometimes more promptly recognized and less difficult to unravel and treat. A young married man, teaching at a college while struggling to complete his Ph.D., was the target for a metabolic disturbance that made him a schizophrenic. For a number of months, he had refused to attend classes—his own, and the ones he taught; and his dissertation was gathering dust on his desk. For a period of four months, he did not leave his room, except to meet his bodily needs; he refused to talk to his wife and friends. He was persuaded to visit an orthomolecular psychiatrist, who, in a series of tests of his blood and urine, found only one possible abnormality. This was a "low normal" blood level of Vitamin B_{12}. The physician gave him a series of intramuscular injections of the vitamin, and after a few weeks of the treatment, the patient broke his silence. He explained that he had retired to his room because his concepts of time and space had become so frighteningly distorted that only within the walls of his bedroom did he feel partially safe. What he described were typical schizophrenic dysperceptions. He had felt himself to be shrinking. Streets appeared to shorten. Time moved in erratic jumps, in which a minute seemed like hours, and hours evaporated in what felt like seconds.

As the vitamin injections were continued, his grasp on reality improved, the dysperceptions faded, and he ultimately was able to return to his studies. His critical need for the vitamin was evidenced by the timing of the injections found essential to keep him normal. If the Vitamin B_{12} was administered every $2\frac{1}{2}$ days, he remained free of symptoms. This being the period required for complete absorption and utilization of the intramuscular injection of the vitamin, it was significant that any lengthening of the interval between shots tended to stir the symptoms again.

The body's utilization of Vitamin B_{12}, which participates in many of its chemistries down to the cellular level, leans on fragile, multi-ordinate mechanisms. The vitamin may not be utilized if the hydrochloric acid level in the stomach is low. Inadequate production of the "intrinsic factor"—a vehicle for absorption of the vitamin, which is needed to convey it through the minute openings in the digestive tract—will cause deficiency in the body even in the face of a generous dietary supply of the factor. Even after the vitamin has penetrated gut openings actually smaller than the molecule of B_{12}, transportation of it may break down, for the body produces two separate vehicles to convey this vital factor to the organs and tissues where it is needed. Any break in the links of that chain will bring with it the consequences of Vitamin B_{12} deficiency, the adequacy of the blood supply notwithstanding. And though physicians were long taught that a lack of Vitamin B_{12} is quickly revealed by the pernicious anemia it causes, the fact is that it may first attack the nervous system and brain, producing psychotic behavior long before the blood displays the tell-tale anemia.

A case illustrating this is the history of an aged woman who, senile, confused, and harboring delusions of persecution, was brought to a psychiatric institution for electric convulsive therapy. The examining physician had a "gut feeling" that her troubles were *not* based, as her family physician thought, on hardening of the arteries (atherosclerosis) of the brain. He sent the elderly woman to a nearby hospital where, in the course of routine tests, they discovered that she was deficient in Vitamin B_{12}. A few injections of this factor brought a sharp recovery. From hindsight, it was obvious that this woman, rather than being a senile dement, confused and paranoid, was the victim of a vitamin deficiency which had attacked her brain and nervous system, and which was entirely responsible for her bizarre behavior, which at one point included her accusation that her husband, innocently bringing the television set nearer her bed for her convenience, was actually trying to irradiate her.

Neither low blood levels of Vitamin B_{12} nor actual psychotic behavior appear in some cases related to the effects of relative deficiency of the vitamin—relative, that is, in terms of an unusually high requirement. A psychiatrist tells of a thirty-eight-year-old woman with a long history of intermittent attacks of severe depression, accompanied by many disabling physical complaints. Psychotherapy had helped, moderately and transiently, but the depressions and her constant fatigue always returned. The Vitamin B_{12} level in her blood, at the time when the physician decided to treat her with the factor, was well within normal range—but what is normal and adequate for one patient may not be for another.

At the time the Vitamin B_{12} therapy was started, the patient was taking several psychotropic drugs—tranquilizers and antidepressants—which took the edge off her acute distress, but still did not allow her to function normally. After the first injection of Vitamin B_{12}, she responded with an increased feeling of well-being and heightened energy reserves, improvements which faded as the effects of the injection wore off. For this reason, the family physician was instructed to repeat the injection every $2\frac{1}{2}$ days. When the patient revisited the psychiatrist, months later, she reported that her energy reserves were much improved, she was less depressed, and her physical complaints were diminishing. With a year of injections at gradually increasing intervals, the patient was able to care for her large family, and to hold down a full time job in a demanding position. Newbold believes this patient has the type of enzyme defect which can be offset by larger than usual supplies of the requisite vitamin. It is a thesis long ago enunciated by Helen Mitchell, who pointed out that we cannot yet supply the needed enzymes when the body's synthesis falls down, but we *can*, with *superdoses* of the nutritional building materials, sometimes encourage the body to manufacture larger amounts of the enzymes. It is ignorance or ignoring of this phenomenon which allows the establishment in nutrition to insist that doses of nutrients "beyond your requirements"—as set by the Washington bureaucracy—are simply wasted. Some people's requirements, because enzyme synthesis differs as much as people themselves do, may not choose to coincide with the modest vitamin-mineral levels on which government agencies have decided to standardize. And while I am voicing that complaint, let me enter another. Are you aware that in many psychiatric hospitals, the Vitamin B_{12} therapy cited in the preceding case history would be frowned on as unorthodox treatment? That is *not* a *theoretical* obstacle to orthomolecular treatment. I can cite the names of the offending institutions and the obstructionist psychiatrists. Their philosophies may explain why it has been estimated that 1 percent of the ''senile'' confined in the sanitaria and institutions could be rescued with injections of Vitamin B_{12}—a simple statement cloaking a major tragedy.

An interesting accomplishment in orthomolecular therapy was reported to me by one of my nutrition students in a course at a community college. She identified herself to me, intriguingly, as ''the porphyrin lady.'' Behind the curious term was a history I quickly identified. Some months before, I had received a call from her physician, seeking possible guidance in any orthomolecular therapy that might spare this patient, who was severely psychotic, from undergoing electric convulsive treatment. He described her symptoms as beginning after her baby was born, with bouts of abdominal pain suggesting a colic associated with gallbladder syndrome; but X rays and other tests revealed no intestinal abnormalities. It would have been tempting, the physician acknowledged, to charge the pains to the psychosomatic, but they were followed by mental confusion which ultimately culminated in severe psychosis. I suggested an examination of her urine for abnormal quantities of porphyrins, which—though the urine had not shown the tell-tale reddish color ordinarily indicating the presence of these factors, and the patient had not displayed the usual sensitivity to light—proved to be there. Therapy with large amounts of B vitamins, desiccated liver, Vitamin C, Vitamin E, and a high protein diet was undertaken. Her appearance at my class was my first report on her progress: she was free of pain and mentally normal. The parallels between this case and the schizophrenias treated with megavitamin doses are closer than they seem. In one type of schizophrenia, of which the Sara syndrome is an aspect, there is a ''mauve'' (pink) spot in the blood, an alien chemical suspected of contributing to psychosis. It has been identified as a pyrrole. Porphyrin is also of that family and is related to, though chemically different from, the type appearing frequently in schizophrenics. Both bear a resemblance to Vitamin B_{12} and to chlorophyll, fascinatingly enough, and both are accused of causing derangements of brain metabolism—of being twisted molecules that contribute to twisted thinking. Pertinent is the appearance of abnormal amounts of porphyrins in the urine of some patients with pellagra, the dietary deficiency disease resulting from insufficient intake of protein and niacin. The psychosis which is one of the symptoms of pellagra bears a resemblance to schizophrenia—a parallel which was the inspiration for Hoffer's use of niacin to treat the latter disease. Incidentally, when the excess porphyrin disappears from the pellagrin's urine, the psychosis fades away, too.

It was many years ago that I first learned that high doses of vitamins and supplements of minerals benefited psychotics. The patient was an elderly woman, who assured me that she had to buy all her food in sealed packages, to be sure that they had not been poisoned by the men she thought were following her. After a few months of the vitamin-mineral supplementing, given for purposes unrelated to her delusions of persecution, she remarked that she could no longer see the men who were following her, but "they're probably hiding around the corner, somewhere." Three months later, when I queried her about her pursuers, she looked at me as if *I* were a little daft, and asked: "What are you talking about?" As one of the pioneers in the philosophy of super-nutrition, I had already taken a beating from my peers, and didn't propose to start a losing battle by reporting a single case. Now the cases run into the many thousands, and the climate is different, but as one psychiatrist remarked to me: "The men who resist this concept will wither on the vine, but as usual, we'll have to wait for them to die, and a new generation to come into practice, acquainted with the truth from the beginning."

I thought of that remark as I read a note passed to me by one of my nutrition students at a university. It read:

"I am sitting in class, comprehending what you're saying, and taking coherent notes. That doesn't sound remarkable until I tell you I was a schizophrenic for eighteen years, fifteen of them spent in one institution after another, and I had more than one-hundred shock treatments. Now, thanks to an open-minded young orthomolecular psychiatrist, I'm well again, and I'll be glad to show you my notes, to prove it."

As gratifying as such a response is in an adult who is a scarred veteran of a decade and a half in institutions, the more so is the response of disturbed children. In each ten thousand children there are three or four who are most abnormal. These autistic and schizophrenic youngsters are the concern of pediatric psychiatrists and psychologists, who have not been able significantly to help them with psychoanalysis or related forms of psychotherapy. Despite the ineffectiveness of these techniques, the large majority of such practitioners cling to them, appearing to surrender to the philosophy of "It's a crooked roulette wheel, but the only one in town."

Dr. Bernard Rimland, a psychologist, was reluctant to accept the claims made for superdoses of vitamins for disturbed children, explaining frankly that his professional training had led him to believe that one's diet contains all the vitamins and minerals required for good nutrition. Persuaded to try the new approach, he confesses now that he has become convinced that his original training and traditional thinking were obviously seriously misguided.

Rimland relates that in the 1960s the press was carrying reports of the orthomolecular treatment of adult schizophrenia with large doses of vitamins. Some of the parents of schizophrenic and of autistic children—either more venturesome or more desperate, or both—undertook on their own the administration of the water-soluble vitamins to their children. Aware that Dr. Rimland and the Institute for Child Behavior Research with which he was affiliated were acting as a clearing house for information, some of these parents wrote to him, reporting the results of their experiments in vitamin therapy for their children. In a period of about two years, he received parental reports from coast to coast, some of which cited significant improvements in the children, as unmistakable responses to the vitamin treatment. What struck Dr. Rimland most forcibly was the curious parallelism in these observations. The parents, independently of each other, were converging on the same vitamins—those which research had linked favorably with the treatment of adult psychoses: niacin, ascorbic acid, pyridoxin (Vitamin B_6), and, less frequently, pantothenic acid. About 50 percent of the reports were favorable, some of the children responding in a degree which, in Dr. Rimland's own word, was "remarkable." His skepticism was undermined by another observation: some of the parents—deliberately or forgetfully—stopped the vitamin dosage, and united in reporting sudden and dramatic regressions in their children's behavior, with an equally sharp improvement when the treatment was resumed. This psychologist's observations confirm those of Cott, another pioneer in these nutritional therapies for autistic, withdrawn, and schizophrenic children, who took joy in the fact that the children, if anything, tended to respond more quickly and more dramatically than the adults.

In the letters from parents, Rimland comments, the most serious universal problem reported was the difficulty parents experienced in finding physicians willing to cooperate in supervising the administration of the vitamins to the young patients. In that observation we see the fruits of the negative attitudes fostered by the philosophies of the F.D.A., the A.M.A., and the policy makers in orthodox psychiatry—many of whom have not treated patients, either by orthodox means or orthomolecular, in many years. Well has it been said, "We tend to be down on what we're not up on."

Typical of reports from mothers of autistic children is this, paraphrased from a letter to an orthomolecular psychologist: "I doubled the pantothenic acid dose, without results. Then I doubled the dose of Vitamin B_6, and this made a distinct difference. My daughter is now very eager to do things—many things, like playing ball, and printing her name and numbers, which she hadn't done for almost a year. The contrast with her previous unwillingness to do anything is unbelievable. Even my husband, who was a disbeliever, says she's improved in just these four days since I doubled the Vitamin B_6 dose.''

The preceding emphasis on the beneficial effect of Vitamin B_6 on the brain will occur again and again in this text. It is a fascinating example of the interplay between nutrients and the chemistry of thinking. One encounters it again, for instance, when an orthomolecular psychiatrist remarks that many schizophrenics do not dream, or do not remember dreaming, until they are given Vitamin B_6, and if the dose is too stimulating, they will complain of excessive dreaming. It is a meaningful observation. Dreams are a necessary outlet for the feelings of a normal person, as Vitamin B_6 is a necessary nutrient which participates in critically important enzyme chemistries of the brain. This is almost an ironic observation, for deficiency of the vitamin, induced by feeding of infants with milk formulas subjected to excessive heat, has been the cause of convulsions, brain damage, and subsequent mental retardation in some babies. One is forced to wonder if the use of formulas in place of beast feeding may not have contributed to autism, to mental retardation considered genetic or congenital, or to schizophrenia of the type suffered by Sara. Vitamin B_6 dependency, involving an inbuilt exaggerated need for the vitamin, has already been linked with a number of disorders involving the brain and nervous systems.

A clear-cut example of B_6 dependency which, unsatisfied, led to psychosis was briefly discussed in the first chapter. The background observations which led to the treatment which rescued a little girl from a mental institution are of themselves fascinating. The history begins with research in diseases of fowl—as far removed from schizophrenia, one would think, as any conceivable scientific investigation could be.

For years, veterinarians struggled with the problem of "perosis," a bone disorder afflicting chickens. They finally found an answer in treatment with Vitamin B_6, zinc, and sometimes, manganese. Little did I dream that the same disorder would one day be reported in human beings, from the same deficiencies; and no one could have persuaded me that the end point of the process might be a type of schizophrenia. By the same token, in publications and broadcasts immediately after World War II, when copper piping came into use, I aroused the wrath of the water industry (and community health departments) by suggesting that the soft water in many areas might pick up excessive amounts of copper, which could be hazardous to the liver and to the nervous system. Again, I didn't envision the possibility that an overload of copper in the body might become a factor in schizophrenia, or that a deficiency of Vitamin B_6, zinc, and manganese in a human being might attack both the bones and the brain. Yet all those entities are involved in the story of Sara, briefly outlined in Chapter One. Her history, reflecting as it does the precise methods by which orthomolecular psychiatry unravels the tangled skein of abnormal molecules which make for twisted emotions and thinking, deserves a complete re-telling.

At the age of eleven, Sara developed knee-joint problems which, in retrospect, bore a marked resemblance to the hock disease and slipped tendon various animal species develop when the diet is deficient in zinc, manganese, and pyridoxin (Vitamin B_6). Her mental troubles also began at age eleven, when she experienced episodes like daydreams—not the normal ones of childhood, but mental voyages far from the world of reality. A few months later, she had lost insight to the point where it was genuinely difficult for her to distinguish between daydream and the real world. At thirteen, she developed chronic insomnia, and began to put on excess weight. In the summer of her fifteenth year, she had the delusion that there was a plot to drive her insane, and there followed the first episode in which she thrashed about, hitting herself—a convulsion her friends believed to be the product of a "bad trip" on LSD (which she actually had not used). Later that year, she attempted suicide by hanging, though she can't recall the attempt and doesn't believe she made it. This was the reason for her first hospitalization. Subsequently, she was transferred to a psychiatric hospital, where her seizures began to occur regularly, at the rate of three a week. Her appetite was poor, and she had episodes of vomiting. Her "therapy," if that term is admissible, consisted of the usual psychiatric hospital techniques, where a few professionals may be charged with treating hundreds of patients: group psychotherapy, tranquilizers, antidepressants, and a drug intended to stop convulsions—which it didn't. In that year, her menstrual cycle stopped.

Two complete neurological studies were done, both pronouncing this psychotic, amnesic, convulsing girl's nervous system and brain to be normal. Thyroid function, urine, and blood chemistries were tested: results, normal. (Please note that the conventional blood tests are called "complete blood chemistries"—CBC, in medical vernacular—which is what they're not, as Sara's later medical history clearly demonstrates.) Sara was then tested psychologically. Intelligent, but not normal. A schizophrenic with paranoid features.

After three months at this psychiatric institution, she was transferred to another. Here an electroencephalogram—a display of her brain waves—was made. Even though traced during one of her seizures, it too, was normal. Now she was treated with a tranquilizer and individual psychotherapy. Results: nothing. At this point, which would have been the prelude to more of the same, with the same lack of results, for the large majority of paranoid schizophrenics, Sara was transferred to still another psychiatric institution where she had her first encounter with orthomolecular testing. Now the blood tests were made for histamine, for factors which are indicators of the metabolism within the cell, and for iron and zinc. These tests revealed abnormalities, but her diagnosis was as yet unchanged. She was a little girl suffering from a seizure disorder which was obviously not epilepsy, since her brain waves were normal and anti-convulsive medications, often used in epilepsy, totally ineffective. And she was a chronic schizophrenic, still under delusions of persecution.

She now transferred to a psychiatric institution where the findings from the orthomolecular tests were reflected in treatment. She was given zinc, manganese, folic acid, pyridoxin, PABA, niacin, Vitamin C, a weekly injection of Vitamin B_{12}, and an antihistamine medication at bedtime. The niacin and Vitamin C doses were gradually increased to three grams daily of each. After only a few days of this treatment, her appetite improved, she was less depressed and had more energy. The improvement was reflected in a new series of blood tests, which also showed changes toward the normal. Two weeks later, group therapy was introduced, and a month later, her psychological testing revealed dramatic improvement, there was further normalization of her blood chemistries and, the most dramatic of all her responses, she had not had a seizure for two weeks. At this point, her family wanted her discharged, since blood tests were now normal and psychological testing showed that she was free of schizophrenic symptoms. At home, the supplements were continued, and with them, the improvement. Her menstrual cycle returned, and became regular. She was free of convulsive episodes for the next two years, without anti-psychotic or anti-epileptic drugs, and her knees—those long neglected indicators of nutritional deficiency—were free of pain.

However, in 1971 Sara developed severe constipation and pain in the spleen area. This was an exacerbation of an old trouble which, like the pain in the knees, had been disregarded because of the pressing need for relief of her mental state and her seizures. This suggested excess excretion of one of the porphyrins, the abnormal chemical to which I referred in the history of the "porphyrin lady." The excess was found, and the researchers also found the "mauve factor" (the pink spot associated with many cases of schizophrenia) to be present. Further, both abnormalities decreased when she took zinc and pyridoxin. The mineral supplements, and the Vitamin B_6 (which was then doubled) proved to be the solution for Sara's troubles, for she is symptom-free with these nutritional aids, though she has been told to increase her intake of the vitamin when she knows that she will be encountering stress.

Dr. Carl Pfeiffer, who led Sara back to normalcy, tells her story in these crisp technical terms:

A case of nutrient deficiency in which vitamins, specifically B_6, and the trace minerals, manganese and zinc were inadequate for the development of normal knee joints and normal brain function. The deficiency, at its peak, was severe enough to cause prolonged psychosis, atypical seizures, arthritis, amenorrhea (absence of the menstrual cycle), constipation, and splenic pain.

Then follows this significant sentence: "The history is given in detail to show the difficulty a patient with a biochemical imbalance may have in seeking treatment." (Establishment—please copy!)

The establishment, instead of heeding, may say that one swallow doesn't make a summer, but of this the psychiatrist-biochemist is well aware. He finishes his technical report with this note:

"After finding the temporary antidote to Sara's illness we have successfully applied these principles of treatment to over 100 problem patients who have the general symptoms of schizophrenia but are unresponsive to anti-psychotic drugs, electroshock, or insulin coma therapy."*

Why "temporary antidote"? Because Sara must continue to use these vitamin-mineral supplements if she wishes to remain symptom-free. Considering that these are harmless and physiological, not alien to the body, it seems a small price to pay for mental and physical normalcy.

As you muse over Sara's history and that of the hundred patients who followed her, perhaps you will recall a statement quoted in Chapter Two, made by a psychiatrist after he cured suicidal depression by removing allergy-causing foods and substances from the patient's environment. He suggested that the case demonstrated what psychiatrists don't know about their patients. Sara, obviously, is another such reminder. Do you suppose that the psychiatrists who plied Sara with the tranquilizers and antidepressants, or leaned on "talking therapy" will, in the light of this little girl's history,

---

*From the case record at the Brain Bio Center, directed by Dr. Pfeiffer.

take a fresh look at what they are doing, and the infrequency of their successes?

Dr. Pfeiffer, based on his experience with schizophrenics with the "Sara syndrome," implicitly warns that blood tests for zinc and vitamin B_6 may reveal levels well within normal range while the patient suffers from deficiency. The "mauve factor" or kryptopyrrole which is produced by these patients under the impact of stress has the capacity to bind the vitamin and mineral in such a way that they are unavailable to the patient, and the only escape from this paradoxical starvation in the midst of adequacy is to saturate the blood with the nutrients, thereby overloading the "binding" capacity and making the Vitamin B_6 and the zinc available to the patient. So exquisitely sensitive is the reaction that a patient like Sara, deprived of the vitamin-mineral supplement for forty-eight hours, will lapse into psychosis. If this seems incredible, consider that chicks hatched from eggs laid by a hen slightly deficient in Vitamin E may turn somersaults backward. Can you imagine how a Freudian avian psychiatrist would regard the veterinarian who would want to treat the chicks with Vitamin E, or give the mother doses to prevent the catastrophe?

The schizophrenics suffering from this metabolic (rather than dietary) deficiency of Vitamin B_6 and zinc have a China-doll or sallow complexion. They suffer from constipation and from pain in the spleen area, and have stretch marks on the thighs, breasts, and hips. Their skin, Pfeiffer reports, refuses to tan and itches on exposure to sunlight—a report doubly fascinating, because the *New York State Journal of Medicine* in the 1950s carried the observation that large doses of Vitamin B_6, taken by individuals abnormally sensitive to sunshine, helped them to avoid burning, blistering, and itching.

These patients are prone to malformation of knee cartilages, and to pain in the knees and other joints. They have white spots on the nails, primarily the result of zinc deficiency, which also causes slow healing of wounds. Morning nausea interferes with their eating breakfast. They are schizophrenics with marked distortions of reality, who don't dream or can't remember dreams—and one of their responses to

Vitamin B_6, if the dose is large enough to overstimulate them, is excessive dreaming. There are neurological symptoms—amnesia, tremor, shaking, and muscle spasms. The men are impotent, the women tend toward irregular or missing menstrual periods. These patients are intolerant of barbiturates. Low blood sugar is frequent, as well as unexplained fever and chills. Anemia of a type responsive only to Vitamin B_6 is present in many patients. So is the mauve factor, with high urinary levels of free kryptopyrrole. Many of the siblings tend to look alike. Not every patient has all these symptoms and signs, but when they distinctly fall into this group perhaps, relative to the schizophrenics whose chemical derangements have not yet been identified, they are fortunate. The biochemical pathway back to normalcy is, for them at least, clearly blazed.

· 4 ·

Children with Biochemical Problems

ON A NATIONAL television program, I was asked about the incidence of low blood sugar. Thinking of the schizophrenics, over 50 percent of whom have hypoglycemia to complicate their problems; and of the disturbed, autistic, brain-damaged, retarded, and hyperactive children who so frequently suffer with it; and of the 15 percent of the "healthy" young draftees who, in Army glucose tolerance tests, proved to have it, I conservatively estimated that about 10 percent of the population suffer with it, intermittently or more or less continually. Dr. Joyce Brothers, a psychologist who was also a guest on the program, commented: "You should be careful not to overdo hypoglycemia, and make it responsible for all mental and emotional disorders." Which is precisely what I had not done, but I said nothing (most rare, for me) because I know that the grizzled male veteran of innumerable scientific debates earns no points in a head-on confrontation with an attractive psychologist.

Had I chosen to reply, I could have reminded Dr. Brothers that *every* study made of patients taking talk-therapy from her profession has shown about 60 percent of them to be victims of hypoglycemia, unrecognized by the practitioners, despite the fact that low blood sugar alone can be responsible for (or intensify) every symptom which brings the patient to the psychiatrist or psychologist. I could also have pointed out, apropos of her warning against sweeping and presumably unjustified claims, that her profession, on the basis of no evidence at all, has burdened millions of American parents, particularly mothers, with the unearned guilt of causing their children's mental and emotional troubles. How many mothers have been unjustly indicted for too little love, for "smother love," or for personally contributing to their children's "oral personality" and the obesity, thumbsucking, cigarette smoking, drug use, or alcoholism supposed to flow from it?

Dr. Brothers' reaction was a subdued version of the fugue into which many of her colleagues are driven when faced with the inescapable realization that the patient has a body—which psychoanalysts explicitly deny—and that it may be adversely affecting the mind. Though our neurology is sophisticated today, man's brain does not yet understand man's brain, or how its nine billion cells really operate. No one genuinely understands how memories are recorded or, for that matter, how association recalls them. No one understands how the emotional aura—good or bad—about a recollection is instantaneously reinvoked, each time it surfaces. No one knows how serendipitous conclusions are formulated (apparently out of the blue, but obviously not), how one group of cells transmits its message to others, how a mere odor brings flashbacks of long-interred memories, why a tranquilizer tranquilizes (or decides to reverse its function, and drive the brain into homicidal rage), why electric convulsive therapy (shock treatment) which leaves behind it no more than small, punctuate hemorrhages in the brain, helps some patients to regain communication, if only fleetingly, with reality; how LSD alters perceptions; why the hallucinations induced by mescaline so intimately resemble those of the schizophrenias; or why elevated blood lactic acid appears to trigger anxiety reactions. Since lactic acid is known to bind (make partially unavailable) the calcium in the blood serum, the orthomolecular physician, instead of prescribing a tranquilizer, may startle his anxiety-ridden patient by canceling the "emotional disturbance" with one or two grams of calcium daily. This may also help to reduce the tendency to muscle spasms which may be based upon the same biochemical aberration; it is also a successful treatment for breath-holding in children, when it is based upon a deficiency of usable calcium in the blood.

All we're sure of is that tranquilizers do generally tranquilize, except when they don't, exactly as nutritionists know, which psychiatrists often don't, that Vitamin E, in some arcane way, dampens the transmission of anxiety impulses from the emotional brain to the thinking brain; but the chemistries remain elusive. Nor do we comprehend why psychiatrists are willing and often eager to prescribe these mind-altering drugs; if they can manage to file their Rx's before the general practitioners beat them to it, but balk at vitamin therapies which, unlike the tranquilizers, have never caused tardive dyskinesia, Parkinson's syndrome, or, in postmenopausal women, breast cancer. Nor do we really know why these experts in the unscience of the mind blame parents for every twist in the psyches of their children, from neurosis to autism to schizophrenia. For if there is one area of firm footing in this quicksand, demonstrable with a few hours spent in any good library, it is this: Parents are not psychic poisons for little people. Bad parents, and bad neighborhoods, and bad companions have produced normal children; good parents have peopled the psychiatric institutions and offices with their progeny. The sour grapes of the parents do not set their children's teeth on edge, but the genes, for which the psychiatrists really shouldn't hold them culpable, may. Added to that, the psychiatrists' understanding of the immutability of heredity is open to challenge too. Heredity *can* be modified. The expression of faulty heredity is deviant biochemistry, and we are learning how to change *that*. Unfortunately, nutrition is here, too, the resource on which we draw, and since nutrients are widely available, harmless, and relatively inexpensive, this approach is not likely to win quick acceptance.

Exactly as physicians study sickness and autopsies—the anatomy of failure—and have little interest in the successes (the living and healthy), so have the men of the mind tended to concentrate on the sick and the abnormal. Pathology spawns thousands of research papers; normalcy attracts neither grants nor research. One of the few papers on the normal in psychology was underwritten by the Air Force a few years ago. They were faced with the problem of explaining, if you please, 100 outstanding officers who appeared to have no psychological problems at all. They sent these oddities to the University of California's Berkeley Counseling Center to find out why they were *not* neurotic, *not* psychotic, *not* emotionally scarred.

The University of California researchers were astonished by their findings. In the backgrounds of these outstanding officers, they found just as much "psychopathology" as one would anticipate in a similar group of male neurotics (and blame for their impairment). There was just as much of mother-hated-father or the reverse; just as much competition with and envy of brothers and sisters; there were just as many broken or stress-filled homes as one would find, and label as the source of psychological warping, in the histories of mentally and emotionally crippled people. And these officers were not only unscarred; they were normal and functioning at an unusually high level. The research is the ultimate comment on a theory which has labeled an untold army of parents as the prime sources of their children's emotional and mental disorders. Psychiatry forgets the resilience of children, as it forgets that a multiplicity of forces act upon the mind (including nutrition, including the body itself).

The study received about as much attention from the talk-oriented profession as one might expect. It was they who, at a meeting at the American Psychiatric Association in 1957, booed Linus Pauling when he predicted that mental illness will ultimately be found, as Freud himself thought, to be essentially biological and biochemical in origin.

With all this, let me here acknowledge the effectiveness with which many therapists—psychiatrists, psychologists, social workers, and perceptive teachers—have helped children with genuine emotional problems. My quarrel is not with a profession, but with the closed minds in a profession which *sui generis* should be open and receptive. I admire the professional who recognizes possible errors in the concepts behind patterning for the brain-injured, but also recognizes the value of the technique. I deplore the psychiatrist who has never tested orthomolecular psychiatry, but knows it won't work, or warns about dangers which have never been demonstrated. And I should like to bar from practice those who treat their patients as if the brain were detached from, had a separate circulation from, and needed a different diet than the body. (I freely confess that in writing these lines, I am thinking of a psychiatrist, a staff member of a state mental hospital who, addressing the anguished father of a severely schizophrenic child, snapped: "I suppose you were too busy with your business to give her any attention." In one sentence, a dogmatic (and unjustified) statement about the origin of schizophrenia, and a gratuitous burden of guilt for a father already reeling under the impact of the illness of a cherished daughter!)

Reluctance to explore the potential of orthomolecular help for troubled children is, of course, another aspect of the notorious cultural lag in medicine, where the interval between a discovery and its application is long enough to become a pit in which millions are trapped and many needlessly suffer and die. In psychiatry, that cultural lag creates the living dead, unable to function and denied the mercy of oblivion. The hyperactive child profits more by megavitamin therapy and fine, additive-free nutrition than by stimulant drugs which may stunt his growth and definitely warp his personality.* The autistic, the withdrawn, the schizophrenic, the retarded, the emotionally deranged, the children suffering from undiagnosed subclinical pellagra masquerading as psychosis, all deserve something less dangerous, more rational, and more genuinely helpful than drugs, and modalities more effective than purely vocal approaches which, as our myriads of distressed parents and waiting lists at institutions testify, are largely bankrupt. Minimal brain damage isn't an explanation,

---

*Amphetamines are poured into hyperactive children as if hyperactivity were caused by an amphetamine deficiency. This is a phenomenon of the American drug culture—both at the level of the public and the medical profession. An English child who is hyperactive is very unlikely to be dosed with such stimulants.

it's a label. Dyslexia is a word, not a concept, not a therapy. "Psychological trauma" is a value judgment which is confronted with opposing *facts*. One of the facts is this: troubled children are casualties of disorders which frequently are biochemical, disturbances which, competently treated with appropriate orthomolecular therapies, can in some cases be harmlessly controlled; in some, completely arrested; in others, cured. There are failures, of course, outnumbered by the successes by a wide margin. Delay in applying such treatment could be the crucial factor in permanently crippling the child, for it is early orthomolecular therapy that yields the best results. Drug therapy is a dangerous kind of palliation, a mask under which the real child struggles to find his identity, through which he tries to perceive the real world. Nutritional therapies are orthomolecular—the right molecule; drugs are malmolecular—the wrong molecule.

The easiest way to dispose of facts that demolish a theory is to challenge them with sophisticated language and concepts. Psychiatrist to parent: "How do you know the child wasn't due for a spontaneous improvement, which would have occurred with or without those vitamins?" (The term for that ploy is "spontaneous remission." It is the first refuge of a psychiatrist whose own therapies have been unproductive for the same child.) A variation on the theme: "How do you know it isn't my previous treatment showing a delayed effect?" A third device: "How do you know it isn't a placebo effect (response to the power of suggestion)?" Does the parent ever stop to realize that an autistic child by definition couldn't possibly respond to the power of suggestion? Isn't it his inability to respond to *anything* other than his private world the mark of the disorder which is the nexus of the problem? And why didn't power of suggestion work with the child when he was previously treated with operant conditioning, injections of steroid hormones or adrenal cortex, patterning, psychotherapy, hypnosis, electric convulsive shock, the talking typewriter, music therapy, and doses of LSD as a garnish to daily intake of virtually every known psychotropic drug? These negative voices remind me of the battle by medical orthodoxy against the introduction of the thermometer as a diagnostic aid. They insisted that people with high fevers were actually cold—didn't they have chills? And who needed the electronic quackery now widely used as the electroencephalograph? And what made Fleming think a mold could produce an antibiotic useful in treating human bacterial infections?

It is constructive to turn, now, and heed the voices of those who are watching children respond to orthomolecular therapies. Here, for instance, are the observations of a psychiatrist who deserted unproductive psychotherapy, for orthomolecular treatment of about 500 children suffering with schizophrenia, autism, brain damage, retardation, learning disabilities, and hyperactivity. The doctor was not an easy convert to the biochemical approach. His training, he has pointed out, had created the belief that one's everyday, average diet contains all the vitamins and minerals one needs, and anyone suggesting the use of large quantities had to be a food faddist, charlatan, or the proprietor of a vitamin business. Then came the realization that a substantial body of evidence had accumulated to show that mentally sick children and adults do, in fact, frequently suffer from markedly abnormal metabolism of such essential nutrients as vitamins, amino acids, and fatty acids. He learned that Dr. Leon Rosenberg of Yale had described nine different diseases which are the result of vitamin dependency, a condition in which the vitamin requirement soars until the gene-dictated requirement far exceeds the supply offered by any conceivable diet. Of these nine disorders, five are responsive to Vitamin B_6, Rosenberg demonstrated. The psychiatrist later was to remark that he has now seen only a few cases of seizures, accompanying schizophrenia or brain-injury in children, which could not be stopped with Vitamin B_6. He read the papers of Pauling, Hoffer, Osmund, and other pioneers, supporting the thesis that high levels of certain vitamins and minerals might overcome the metabolic derangements characteristic of many forms of mental illness. He could not ignore, for instance, the report by two psychiatrists that eleven of a group of nineteen psychotic children displayed an abnormality of protein (tryptophane) metabolism which could be corrected with supplements of Vitamin B_6, provided the dose was twenty times the amount set by the F.D.A. as the "Recommended Dietary Allowance" for children. (The psychiatrist shortly learned from experience that doses up to two hundred times that standard benefited many disturbed children.) Similar well-documented reports appeared on Vitamin C and on niacin. With the latter vitamin, the obstructionists again leaped into the arena, proclaiming that niacin cures the insanity caused by pellagra only because the disease is caused by lack of the vitamin. A person with a normal diet, they insisted, gets enough niacin to prevent mental disease, and additional amounts would do nothing. The psychiatrist closed his ears to the professional orthodoxy, and applied niacin treatment for problem children. They not only responded, but their improvement, he happily reported, was more dramatic than in adults. He was now induced by the response to try the therapy for autism, considering that this childhood disorder, too, was the result of a metabolic error, and that the overlapping of the symptoms of the two sicknesses reflected distortions of perception, caused by deficiencies of vitamin-dependent enzymes in the cells of the brain, with accumulation of toxic (and, quite logically) hallucinogenic substances in the bloodstream.

Even when these autistic children can't communicate, there is objective evidence that such perceptual distortions exist for them, and make their private worlds a Dantesque hell. They suffer from strange aberrations in perception of time, space, depth, vision, hearing, and their images of their own bodies. An autistic child is described by the psychiatrist as lifting his foot very high when stepping from the bare floor to a carpeted area, as though he perceived the carpet as being a foot high. Parents commented to him on the great fear the children exhibited in descending a flight of stairs, with none in ascending them. The psychiatrist guesses that the bottom of the staircase would seem to autistic children as receding endlessly and frighteningly into the distance. Other symptoms bespeak a twisting of reality: their poor balance, frequent falling, walking in a zigzag fashion, bumping into objects, walking on tiptoe while peering anxiously at the floor. We readily accept such distortions as being produced by the impact of hallucinogenic drugs on the brain, as we accept the imaginary pink elephants of the alcoholic with delirium tremens (a disorder long ago treated successfully with megavitamin therapy). Why should there be such hostility to the concept of dysperception caused by hallucinogenic chemicals manufactured by the body itself, as a product of biochemical disturbances for which there is both objective evidence and a sound theoretical base? And, with consideration of the potent and harmful drugs prescribed for these children in an effort unphysiologically to change brain chemistry, why the reluctance to use harmless nutrients, normal to the organism, in the attempt to correct the metabolic error?

An orthomolecular psychiatrist who read this manuscript said, vis-à-vis the preceding paragraph: "They'll all be on this bandwagon in ten years, or they won't be practicing."

Apropos of distortions of reality based on metabolic disturbances which are correctible with a nutrient, ask any competent nutritionist. He will cite the elderly, confused, aggressive, paranoid "senile dement" who is neither senile nor in the classical sense demented, but a victim of a Vitamin B_{12} deficiency which has attacked the nervous system and the brain, with no evidence of the pernicious anemia it ordinarily causes. The result is senile behavior with overtones of delusions of persecution, all stemming from the changes of body chemistry derived from lack of a daily amount of Vitamin B_{12} weighing less than a period made with a lead pencil.

To come back to the child psychiatrist—he spells out his observations of the improvements he watched in some of his young patients: the child, he writes, begins to comprehend and obey commands—a small gain, if you have never seen an autistic child, a small miracle, if you have. The youngster shows, for the first time, a willingness and an ability to cooperate with his parents and others. Hyperactivity in disturbed children subsides slowly in many cases; in others, it stops or is dramatically reduced in one or two weeks of treatment. Gaze aversion—the unwillingness of these children to look one in the eye—fades away. Affection is accepted and returned.

Apropos of the influence of the power of suggestion, the practitioner has observed cases where children responded to the treatment, and then, for one reason or another, were deprived of part or all the dose, or could not retain it because of nausea caused by a virus infection. These children reverted, sometimes within a few days, to their hyperactivity, withdrawal, muteness, screaming, or non-communication, which should, except for opponents who are exquisitely sensitive to their own suggestions, dispose of the placebo effect. If additional evidence is needed, there are the observations, previously cited, linking food additives to many cases of hyperactivity. Withdrawal of the additives brings improvement in the children; restoring the chemicals to the diet—without the children's knowledge—reignites the symptoms. Rimland's studies also supply evidence of the effectiveness of the orthomolecular therapies for the autistic for, with the cooperation of the parents, there was a deliberate on-off schedule in which the vitamins were discontinued periodically. After ten days of non-treatment for a child who had shown a favorable response to the vitamins, a mother wrote to Dr. Rimland: "He seems to have withdrawn into himself, no longer exhibiting the lively interest in the world around him that had marked the previous month." She added that his new-found willingness to cooperate and obey such directions as he understood, disappeared rapidly, and his old mannerisms, bizarre hand motions and positions, which had been waning, reasserted themselves "with a vengeance."

Do they hold their gains? A psychiatrist writes about a badly disturbed child who was given orthomolecular treatment for seven months, after which he was well enough to be withdrawn from a special school, and to attend one for normal children. Another young patient, after treatment for two years, became well enough to return home from school on his own, use his key to admit himself, and watch TV or otherwise amuse himself until his mother, who is employed, returns about a half hour later. I personally have seen a somewhat retarded, brain-injured child, whose nutritional treatment I formulated for her pediatrician, gain enough ground during a single summer to transfer to a class for normal children in the fall, but I must emphasize that only about half the children treated in the orthomolecular way show a response; and not all who respond do so as significantly as we hope for. About 3 percent of the autistic children in the Rimland studies could not tolerate the nutritional treatment, and, while it did no harm, it had to be withdrawn. Autism, obviously, is a single term covering more than one disorder. We are still left with gain never achieved by talk therapy, devotion, punishment, or tranquilizers and other psychotropic medication.

A child need not be autistic or schizophrenic to suffer with dysperceptions. There are other and less complex causes, which may go unrecognized. Some of these children may erroneously be considered slow learners or victims of difficulties based on brain damage. Behind these descriptions may be a very different entity: inbuilt, unsatisfied elevated needs for certain nutrients. For example, there is the story of a quiet, sad little boy, eleven years old, who came to a general practitioner's office for treatment of a sore throat. Thorough examination revealed no reason for soreness, nor any for his apparent dejection. The child, speaking so softly as to be almost inaudible, finally admitted that he was depressed because for almost a year he had experienced difficult in reading. Pressed for details, he said the words seemed to move on the page, numbers reversed (86 became 68), people's sizes altered, and there appeared to be a bright light about them. His hands also appeared to change size—usually becoming larger; he felt tired most of the time, and he couldn't sleep soundly. Sometimes, as he looked at a word, letters would disappear: *silly* became *sill*, *tent* looked like *ten*. As you will learn, it takes an experienced practitioner to elicit such admissions from a child, explaining why the ''slow learning,'' gradually appearing in a student formerly considered average

or even bright, is often unrecognized as a symptom of dysperception.

The physician prescribed a gram of niacin (1,000 mgs.)
and a gram of Vitamin C after each meal, three times daily
and, aware of the poor dietary history he finds in the poverty
area in which he practices, urged the child to eat more protein—meat, particularly. When he returned to the doctor, six
weeks later, he reported that the disturbing changes in the
size of his hands and in people had disappeared, he was
sleeping better, and the imaginary voices he had been hearing
had become less frequent. A year later, he wrote a grateful
letter to his physician, to tell him that the things he used to
see and feel weren't bothering him any more. He said that
he was no longer forgetful or drowsy, but feeling and thinking
better. He boasted that he had more friends, and that his
school marks had doubled (he felt he could bring them even
higher). "I thank you," he closed his letter, "for helping me
out with these problems." A year later, the doctor reexam-
ined him, and pronounced him normal. His small patient had
become captain of the school soccer team. What would he
have become if the diagnosis had been schizophrenia, because of the perceptual distortions and the depression, and
the physician had been an analyst, and the treatment had been
psychotropic medication and a probing of the child's traumatic experiences in toilet training?

The terror unleashed by a *suddenly* unstable universe, in
which objects move or change size, may prevent a child from
discussing his problem, even with peers, parents, or physician. If the symptoms arise gradually, the child may be somewhat unaware of the extent to which his concepts of himself
and the real world about him are distorted. Even older children may be reluctant to discuss what is happening to them.
I recall a teenager who approached me after my lecture on
orthomolecular concepts and talked about her "nervousness," which was an understatement for the atmosphere about
her of a ticking bomb. She said that her mother and her psychiatrist considered her to be a delinquent, rather than a sick
young woman. About her was a mouse-like odor, familiar to

anyone who has spent enough time with enough schizophrenics. Her face was strikingly pale, a phenomenon I have observed in schizophrenics who are experiencing auditory hallucinations—the voices that aren't really there. I asked her about the voices, and her reply was another interesting commentary on what psychiatrists do not know about their patients. "Oh, God," she said, apparently convinced that I alone in her world could hear them too, "I never even told my shrink about them." Her psychiatrist had threatened her with shock treatment, she said, if she didn't stop misbehaving—as if she could. After our conversation, she traveled hundreds of miles to consult a medical nutritionist, there being no orthomolecular psychiatrist anywhere in the area. A year later, after treatment with niacin, Deaner, B_6, C, E, zinc, manganese, and mild doses of the tranquilizer she had previously used, she was back in school, functioning well, and minus what she called "the orchestra in my head."

Since the delusion of the moving of letters and numbers is a common symptom of an unsatisfied need for niacin (and other nutrients) it is important to identify it. To the child, it may seem that the words on the blackboard or page move up and down or sideways. Sometimes they seem to move off the page or board, and may or may not return, and the children can't describe how they are able to "trap" and read them. For some children, the words appear to move close, away, and close again, as though their eyes were zoom lenses. Often the child will say that the words appear with a "ghost image," a shadow or a doubling, which appears to be analogous to the doubling of a television picture when the signal is partially bounced off an obstruction in its path. In severe cases the letters are unaligned or even reversed. Doubling is not the extreme of the symptom; one physician worked with a child who saw a single word appear *five* times in a vertical row. Occasionally the words or figures become so distorted that the children can't recognize them—to one youngster, asked to look at the number "69" and draw it, it obviously appeared to resemble the outline of a pair of human ears. When children are struggling with these distortions of perception, they will try to memorize what they are told, so that they will be able to feed back to the teachers what is desired, even though they are not seeing what the teachers think they are. Under such circumstances, the child's success in school will obviously be in inverse proportion to the intensity of his dysperceptions, and one must sympathize with children who are tortured in the academic process as their brains react to input which in no way reflects the real world.

Another history of a little girl illustrates that the disturbance in the molecular environment of the brain, however devastating its impact on perception and function, may sometimes be relatively simple to correct. The eleven-year-old was in the physician's office for treatment for abdominal pains and headaches, for which the practitioner could find no physical base. Formerly an excellent student and a pleasant child, she was obviously worried about failing in her school work, and highly irritable. Instead of dismissing the symptoms as psychosomatic, the physician explored the possibility of the somato-psychic, which is, of course, the influence of body on mind. He asked her the key questions that confirm the dysperceptions characteristic of subclinical pellagra. Do words on the blackboard seem to move? Does your face in the mirror seem to grow larger and smaller? (The words did move; her face changed size, but then so did the faces of other members of her family.) Do you hear voices that aren't really there, calling your name? (She did—they invited her out to play.) Do foods taste strange? (So strange she preferred not to eat.) Was this early schizophrenia? To this physician, the term is meaningless, and a stigma, at that. Metabolic dysperception would be closer to the reality, but the concept of perceptual distortion based on disturbances of cerebral chemistry would be incomprehensible to the average layman, and medical insurance carriers would probably reject it. However, pellagra is, in its impact on the mind, somewhat parallel to schizophrenia, and it is a vitamin deficiency disease, much more acceptable a concept to the layman. Even when the vitamin deficiency is only in relation to an unusually high requirement, it is easier for the family to accept than a mental disorder. Likewise, the insurance people are happier and, while other doctors may scoff, the patient is happier too, for with large doses of niacin, Vitamin C, pyridoxin, Vitamin E, a natural source of the Vitamin B complex (such as dried liver) and an improved diet, the symptoms gradually leave. In the case of the little girl, the doctor used only niacin and Vitamin C, and he comments: "The change in two weeks was remarkable; in a month, even more so." In the light of his experience with a large practice in an economically depressed area, he has found that 5 to 10 percent of the patients he treats suffer with perceptual dysfunction which responds to niacin—i.e., pellagra affecting only the brain, minus the skin rash and the diarrhea considered to be (with psychosis) the classic symptoms of that severe deficiency disease. He obviously agrees that Linus Pauling: a deficiency disease may choose to strike only one target in the body. Pellagra affecting only the brain does exist. The interesting aspect of this "new" theory is the fact that it is neither new nor a theory. Tom Spies, the great medical nutritionist, demonstrated more than three decades ago that mild mental disturbances are inevitably the early price for chronic, mild deficiency in niacin. Among those symptoms, as I listed them in a book I wrote in 1940, were nervousness, sensitivity to noise, crying with little or no provocation, severe and unprovoked anxiety, insomnia, and—to quote that long-ago book—"imagining things—someone coming up to the walk, someone calling them, someone in the room . . . melancholia without knowing why. . . . " While Pellagra ordinarily strikes brain, skin, and digestive tract—hence, the disease of the three "D's"—diarrhea, dermatitis, delirium—it may choose to affect only the brain. I may add a personal observation to emphasize that truth. Not only does cerebral pellagra exist, but when the vitamin deficiency is both mild and chronic, its symptoms may not be those of psychosis. They could be mistaken for neurosis, or they may not be susceptible of any pat label—the price may be just dull thinking and mental confusion.

Who develops such a deficiency? The doctor gives the answers arising from his intensive study of his patients and their families. It occurs in people who eat low-protein diets, linked with vitamin deficiency because the body manufacturers two vitamins from protein (amino acids). It tends to run in families—which may be because of communal menus or communal genes. It responds to vitamin treatment if it is diagnosed early and promptly treated. He suspects that many teenagers suffer from it, too, which is ironic when we remember that the early research, fifty years ago, which led us to recognize niacin as a factor needed to prevent pellagra, was performed with convicts as volunteer subjects. He regards bed-wetting in children as a possible sign of it, particularly when they also complain that they can't see the blackboard, and that a new prescription for glasses is unhelpful. Sleeping poorly, when linked with the other symptoms, tends to confirm the diagnosis. The doctor implicates the high carbohydrate diet, which is, of course, the corollary of low-protein. This is to say that people who won't eat or can't afford to eat meat, eggs, and other high protein foods are likely to fill themselves with cheap starches and sugars. Many of these patients are saturated with sugar, as schizophrenic patients often are. For this reason, the doctor puts them on the hypoglycemia diet, high in protein, low in starch, as free of sugar as possible. (He is wise in doing so, if only because of three common symptoms caused by hypoglycemia: a feeling of being detached from reality, sometimes expressed as "I feel like two people in one body, one watching the other"; difficulty with the concentration and memory spans; and pronounced irritability.)

A New York psychiatrist has also come to the firm conclusion, after orthomolecular treatment of hundreds of schizophrenic and autistic children, that the approach shows greater promise than any other that has been tried. He places great emphasis on Vitamin B_6, as do practically all workers in this field, uses niacin or niacinamide, Vitamin C, and calcium pantothenate. Not only has he reported control of hyperactivity, increased interest in learning, and ability to give and receive emotion, but, in the brain-injured, strikingly quick relief from seizures (convulsions). He quotes parents who, eleven days after starting their brain-injured child on Vitamin B$_6$, joyfully reported that their son had experienced his first seizure-free day in three years—years in which, without effect, he had been heavily dosed with phenobarbital and antiepilepsy medications. Another child, who had had multiple daily seizures for two years, became free of them while receiving megavitamin treatment, and has remained free to date (four years). I don't wish to belabor the inconsistencies of the profession, but it is relevant that at least one of the antiepilepsy drugs commonly used *causes* severe vitamin deficiency, as *one* of its side effects; yet the practitioners who prescribe these do not, in my experience, accept the megavitamin therapy as a viable theory. Vitamin deficiency, yes; vitamin therapy, no!

If while reading of the dividends children with seizures obtain from large doses of Vitamin B$_6$, you comfortably assume that a deficiency in the vitamin is a threat to everyone's child but yours, you might consider the following facts:

The Vitamin B$_6$ content of the foods that comprise half our diet, in terms of calorie contributions, has been reduced about 80 percent. That takes in sugar and all white flour products, including bread, cookies, cakes, tarts, sugar, spaghetti and macaroni, cereals, and all the overprocessed grains which 94 percent of the public choose, such as wheat, rye, barley, corn, and rice.

The baby fed on formula is cheated in two ways: while cow's milk supplies about as much Vitamin B$_6$ as mother's milk, the cow's milk is diluted with considerable amounts of water, and is modified with a processed carbohydrate that does not supply Vitamin B$_6$. Second, mother's milk isn't sterilized at high heat, as prepared formulas are—and the formulas are reheated by mother and, sometimes, reheated twice. The effect of this may be to bind the Vitamin B$_6$ so that it is less available to the baby's metabolism. In fact, when baby formulas were sold in ordinary tin cans which were not internally lined with a resin, the tin of the can reacted with the Vitamin B$_6$, totally binding it. The price for that processing technique was hundreds of babies with convulsions, some of whom became brain-damaged, and at least one of whom now has an I.Q. at the idiocy level.

Your pediatrician has been assured by the A.M.A. that babies need only extra Vitamin A and D. The A.M.A. is not worried about Vitamin B_6. Those who are, are described as food faddists. When the child so neglected develops convulsions for which Vitamin B_6 supplements prove to be therapeutic, that is no longer food faddism, but a triumph of modern medicine. When Vitamin B_6 is used, with other nutrients, to treat autism or childhood schizophrenia, you are flirting with unorthodox medicine.

Dietary taboos are sometimes as effective as food supplements in treating mental and emotional ills, both in children and adults. At the University of Pennsylvania, Dr. F. Curtis Dohan, Professor of Medicine, demonstrated that diets free of gluten (wheat protein) improved the behavior of schizophrenic patients to a degree which allowed their release from the locked wards. Cott remarks on the same phenomenon with children: parents have reported rapid and dramatic improvement in hyperactive children following the use of the hypoglycemia diet, which severely limits starch, and avoids sugar as much as possible. The use of a hypoglycemia diet completely free of wheat is more effective for some patients. I have pointed out that our institutional psychiatrists and dietitians have obviously not read Dohan's papers, or have chosen to ignore their findings, despite the fact that they simply confirm what was observed in Europe during World War II, when wheat imports were reduced by 50 percent and schizophrenic admissions to the mental hospitals fell by nearly the same percentage. On Formosa, natives eating very little of the grains are reported to have a schizophrenic rate nearly two-thirds less than that of Northern Europe. How many institutionalized schizophrenics might be improving or released to rejoin society, if bread were not the staff of mental hospital diets, because it's cheaper? It becomes obvious that overprocessed grains may be a double barreled threat to mentally troubled children and adults. The gluten may act as a toxin. The loss of Vitamin B_6 in the highly processed grains is a significant threat to brain function, particularly to victims of the Sara syndrome and to the brain-injured children who are subject to seizures.

Before your memory of Chapter Two fades, you should be reminded that allergic symptoms may intensify or masquerade as psychiatric troubles in children. Consider the ten-year-old girl who staggered out of a school lavatory, so confused and behaving so bizarrely that her teachers suspected her of taking drugs. That reaction was caused specifically by exposure to a disinfectant which had been used in the toilet. Similar reactions were created when the child was exposed to the solvents in a felt-tipped pen and that evaporating from freshly mimeographed paper. When the allergist exposed her to solvents, the patient developed a psychotic reaction which lasted three hours, regressing to infantile behavior, mistaking her mother for a male school teacher in whose class she had been two years previously, and seeing the physician's face as purple spots floating on a yellow background. She remembered nothing of the episode, recalling only that she had initially become dizzy and sleepy. Treatment by the allergist, with hyposensitization and removal of offending substances from her environment created a striking improvement in the child's mental health. The allergist has since helped more than 200 patients with psychic symptoms by eliminating allergens from their diets and environments, but he has been driven to wonder, as he phrased it: "Would it not be a shame if such persons where confined to mental institutions, some of them perhaps even in catatonic states, being fed through stomach tubes with the very food to which they are allergic?" We may reasonably conclude that examination of troubled children for allergies and for hypoglycemia—which you now know to be interrelated—may be a rewarding step in helping them toward normalcy.

Although Cott, other researchers, and I estimate that about 10 percent of the non-schizophrenic population has hypoglycemia, at least 50 percent of the schizophrenics do, and in some reports, not only is the estimated percentage higher, but the low blood sugar is regarded as part of the schizophrenic process. The diet self-chosen by schizophrenics before and during their illness is that which places a burden upon the adrenal glands, stress on which has been accused of contributing to mental disease: sweets, candy, cakes, doughnuts, coffee, tea, chocolate, cola and other soft drinks. The role of the sugar and caffeine in such a diet in causing low blood sugar, plus its deficits in protein, vitamins and minerals, are explained in Section II, where you will realize that the condition is often not recognized because of failure to test for it, failure to administer the test properly, incompetent interpretation of the results, or failure to evaluate other factors which may disturb the equilibrium of sugar metabolism in the body. Suffice it here to say that a test which reveals diabetes may not reveal the corollary disease: hypoglycemia; and the conventional (and competent) test for hypoglycemia may fail to reveal allergies which are causing the condition or resulting from it.

To give a hypothetical example (and one frequently observed by the psychonutritionist who tests for neuroallergy), we may see a child or adult who shows good but limited improvement when placed on the hypoglycemia diet. The plateau of improvement may be pierced, and added gains achieved by withdrawal from the diet of good—but allergenic—foods to which he is sensitive. If withdrawal of wheat produces added benefits, the role of the grain in causing troubles for the child is accurately defined, harmlessly and inexpensively. Exclusion of milk would be tested in the same way. Allergies to petrochemicals, molds, and other foods would, for the most part, require testing by an allergist, though there is a home method of identifying some food allergies by noting the rise in the pulse rate after ingestion of foods, consumed one at a time. If the pulse rises more than eighteen beats, or reaches more than eighty-four per minute (whether or not that reflects a rise of eighteen or more beats) allergy to the food is probable. Interested readers may consult Dr. Arthur Coca's book on the pulse rate test for allergy.

It is obvious from what you have read that the orthomolecular treatment is multi-faceted, and usually comprises much more than a dose of this vitamin or that mineral. Yet the unilateral approach of a dose of one vitamin is the method employed in many of the tests the talk-tranquilizer-therapists have conducted to "prove" the method doesn't work. It would be instructive for them (and you) to follow a little boy through his sickness and his treatment by an orthomolecular psychiatrist. Although Bob was only twelve, he was a veteran of innumerable sessions with child psychiatrists, psychotherapists, and social workers. The diagnoses were uniformly polysyllabic but never in agreement, from one professional office to another, and the tranquilizers (and doses of them) prescribed seldom coincided, and the psychological approaches varied with each practitioner, but the results were the same: Bob was very sick, and becoming sicker. He heard voices which said bad things about him, these including the voice of his father (who had been dead for five years), and those of his brother and some of his schoolmates—when he was alone. He had been picked up for shoplifting, in stores where he usually stole chocolate bars, his consumption of which sometimes reached over three pounds in one day. Bob had, without provocation, physically attacked his mother, his brother, and several fellow students. In the classroom, he alternated between staring, with his eyes obviously out of focus, and sleeping, with his head on the desk. Several times, at school and at home, he set fires.

Those who had treated Bob had made no tests of his chemistries; none of them paid the slightest attention to his pathological sweet tooth, though that is one of the most common symptoms of low blood sugar, and hypoglycemia is fully capable of re-enforcing, if not initiating, symptoms like Bob's. Nonetheless, a number of these psychiatrists had recommended that the proper place for Bob was in an institution. Electric convulsive therapy had been strongly suggested, too, interestingly, by the same professional who told the family that megavitamin therapy was (a) ineffective, and (b) somehow possibly dangerous. I might note here that electric convulsive therapy (shock) is not without its dangers, and in many cases it yields no benefits at all, does harm, or produces improvements which are transient. Sometimes, when it is combined with orthomolecular treatment, the forecast for it is considerably better.

In Bob's case, the orthomolecular psychiatrist, more than suspicious of low blood sugar, ordered the standard glucose tolerance test for the child. It revealed a severe hypoglycemia, a result inevitable in view of his insatiable appetite for sweets, which had to mean that he was burning sugar faster than he could replace it. Blood, liver, and glandular tests revealed nothing significant. Urine and hair tests showed some abnormalities of a type frequent in hypoglycemics.

The child was placed on the hypoglycemia diet. With each meal, he took substantial amounts of niacin, Vitamin C, B_6, E, and a multiple vitamin supplement. To provide the between-meal high protein snacks helpful in keeping the blood sugar at a level which would permit Bob's brain and nervous system to function properly, he was provided with concentrated protein tablets. The school nurse and the teachers were drafted to make sure the child took them, didn't buy sweets, and wasn't being supplied with candy by his few friends. These measures are sometimes necessary in the early stages of the treatment of hypoglycemia, when the craving for sweets may induce cheating. As the treatment goes on, in most cases the sweet tooth gradually diminishes, and may disappear.

Bob didn't recover overnight, nor were there miraculous changes in the first few months. He grew calmer in that period, and related better to his brother and his schoolmates. Gradually, his attention span and ability to concentrate improved, and his sleeping bettered. No attacks on his family or his fellow students occurred after the therapy started. Though on the hypoglycemia diet he was allowed generous amounts of protein and fat, the boy lost some of his excess weight. In the first few months, he still occasionally clashed with his mother, argued bitterly with his brother, and, on several occasions, created an uproar in the classroom, but this behavior faded away, and by the end of the fourth month of treatment, it was obvious that his perceptual distortions were gone, that he no longer had delusions about conversations with his deceased father, and heard no more imaginary voices. Occasionally his craving for sweets reappeared and led him to cheat, but he himself came to recognize the toll for deviations from the prescribed diet. He once remarked to the psychiatrist: "I got detention at school today, but that was because I had a Coke, and didn't know how to stop what I was doing." The caffeine and sugar of the soft drink took only forty-five minutes to start Bob on a classroom rampage.

What does the future hold for the little boy? He is no longer schizophrenic, by any of the tests that sensitively measure the symptoms of those disorders, nor by the standard of his every day behavior. He may be an arrested schizophrenic, but in any case, he will take his supplements of vitamins for at least five years, with his dosage gradually lowered if his progress warrants that. Ultimately, the psychiatrist will totally withdraw the megavitamins, to see if Bob can hold his gains. He will, however, keep the child on the low carbohydrate diet indefinitely, for hypoglycemia is not cured, but arrested, and is capable of flaring up if Bob tries to return to the sugar-saturated foods of average Americans. If the hypoglycemia is again touched off, it will announce its presence plainly, for it can bring on symptoms indistinguishable from those of severe neurosis or of psychosis.

Were it not for the dedicated, expert, and advanced care the child received, Bob today would at best be a dweller on the fringe, of but not in society. At worst, which is where he was heading, and, indeed, had been referred by his previous physicians, he would be another cipher in the growing population of children in homes for the seriously disturbed. Not all Bobs respond to the biochemical-nutritional approach, and only a minority do so in a few months, but authorities estimate that 80 percent of *all* schizophrenics who receive orthomolecular therapy *early* in the progress of the disease can be returned to normal function, and, even more important, with a striking reduction in the percentage of those who, treated by the outmoded methods, would inevitably suffer new attacks and be forced to return to the institutions.

The skepticism of psychiatrists is often equalled by that of the general practitioner or pediatrician, but occasionally the medical man is driven into enthusiasm for the new approach. Rimland, whom I have previously quoted, created a special vitamin formula for autistic children, based on the four vitamins reported by parents to be helpful in their own medically unsupervised treatment of their afflicted children. (These were niacinamide, pantothenic acid, pyridoxin, and Vitamin C.) The Rimland staff enrolled some 300 autistic children in a nation-wide study, but parents of the participating children were required to obtain medical supervision, which promptly created conflicts with disbelieving physicians. One doctor, Rimland notes, was positive that the parents of two autistic children were victims of a swindle in the proposed study, and wrote to Dr. Linus Pauling, who had agreed to respond personally to any physician querying the validity and concerned about the safety of the megavitamin research program. The personal reply from Dr. Pauling won the physician's reluctant consent to the children's taking part in the study. The children responded to the vitamins to such a degree that the once-skeptical physician wrote to Dr. Rimland, to ask if the family's other three children, who had learning disabilities, could be enrolled in the research project. He had good reasons: the two autistic brothers had, like some other children in the study, responded with reduced tantrums, increased alertness, better patterns of sleep, greater sociability, and improved speech. Failures in the Rimland study, it goes without saying, occurred, in part because autism, like the schizophrenias, is not one disease. For instance, youngsters whose behavior was altered by destruction of brain tissue by a viral infection, Rimland remarks, would not respond. But the computer showed that well over 50 percent of the children *did,* some of them dramatically. One mother, whose daughter had shown no significant response to the basic vitamin dosages, followed instructions to double the Vitamin B_6 dose for her daughter, and wrote excitedly to tell the researchers that her daughter had shown great improvement on the doubled Vitamin B_6 intake. She described her as intellectually sharper, more aware of the outside world, and, for the very first time, participating in a Hebrew holiday ritual by singing a song "from beginning to end."

Although Rimland observed that children suffering from viral destruction of brain tissue were among those who did not respond to the megavitamin treatment, it should not be thought that we have no nutritional resources for children in these special categories. In spastics with cerebral palsy, in postviral encephalitic syndrome, and in other disorders involving brain damage, we in nutrition have made progress which contradicts the dicta of neurologists, who were taught that cerebral nerve cells cannot be repaired. I have observed evidence of such repair, following administration of a 27-carbon waxy, long chain alcohol, concentrated from wheat germ oil. Its presence in wheat germ oil may explain the persistent reports of its usefulness in the adjunct treatment of cerebral palsy, and multiple sclerosis and other myoneuropathies (nerve-muscle disorders). When I discussed this research with Dr. Andrew Ivy, one of the great physiologists of our time, he indicated that he has unpublished work in his laboratory indicating that the neurology textbooks are in error in insisting that damaged cerebral neurones are beyond repair. (I have called this research to Dr. Rimland's attention.)

Other nutritional factors sometimes fly to a specific target. That was reemphasized when the Rimland group, at the urging of my departed friend, Adelle Davis, added magnesium to the supplements. She had advised them to do so when the study was initiated, but the researchers hesitated to add still another handful of pills to the formidable list. Adelle had warned them that the need for magnesium would be increased by the administration of Vitamin B$_6$, for lack of which mineral the children would encounter problems in bedwetting, sound sensitivity, and irritability. Dr. Rimland remarks that she predicted exactly what happened with one group of the children in the study.

In conversation with Dr. Carl Pfeiffer at the Brain Bio Center where he identified and successfully treated the Sara syndrome, and where I met the heroine of this medical saga, I used the familiar term "mentally retarded," and was chided by the medical biochemist. "Mentally dormant," he suggested, was a more realistic term. It was obvious that his research in orthomolecular treatment for such children had yielded dividends suggesting that their potential is well beyond what we have thought it to be. Certainly that conclusion is reenforced if you read the publications by Dr. Henry Turkel, who demonstrated in words, photographs, and X rays that the "slow motion picture of a normal child" which is the mongoloid can be spurred into maturation. Despite the voluminous evidence Dr. Turkel presents, he has encountered vicious obstructionism from the Food and Drug Administration, whose hostility toward any therapeutic claims for vitamins has been delineated and deplored before Congressional and Senate committees and, indeed, in speeches in both houses of Congress. I do not propose here to review the Turkel method of treatment of mongoloids; it is not only complex, involving both nutrients and drugs, but it often must be individualized for each patient. The full details are available in Dr. Turkel's text: *New Hope for the Mentally Retarded— Stymied by the F.D.A.*, published by Vantage Press. I do want to asseverate this researcher's claim that mongoloids can be stimulated into both physical and mental progress beyond any level that has been achieved by older methods, for I have seen responses in these children to megavitamin and other orthomolecular treatments, long before these terms were used for such therapies. I refer your physician to the Turkel text, and to future publications by Dr. Carl Pfeiffer, for I am sure that his cryptic remark about "mentally dormant" as a better term than "mentally retarded" refers to research which he will one day publish.

Returning to conventional psychotherapy for a moment, let us remember that patients subjected to a great deal of it become dependent upon it, whether or not it is helpful. The orthomolecular psychiatrist must be prepared to continue such sessions, at least in the early stages of the biochemical treatment, for such "psychology-addicted" patients have the greatest reluctance in accepting the fact that their illnesses have a physical basis, and can be kept motivated into following the regime faithfully only with support and encouragement from the practitioner and from the family. A tranquilizer is often helpful in the first few months for, as I observed earlier, the schizophrenics are likely to complain, "Those vitamins are turning my brain upside down!" and react with increased nervousness, for a while. Their statement is true, but misworded: their brains are being turned right side up. Some patients will need help beyond a tranquilizer, vitamins, minerals, and a hypoglycemia diet, and there *are* many ways in which the regime can profitably be modified to meet the individual needs of the children.

Other than threats of toxicities never demonstrated, the psychotherapists sometimes employ what Dr. Harvey Ross has called psychological blackmail. It is an apt term for those who warn their child patients that they will not continue to see them, if they start orthomolecular treatment. It is not an uncommon reaction for professionals who feel threatened by a new modality. I once heard a cardiologist tell an aged patient, himself a physician, who had covertly taken and profited by, Vitamin E for his heart trouble, that any of his patients who took Vitamin E for heart disease would have to find another heart specialist. This while he was looking at an electrocardiogram reflecting improvement he *knew* his digitalis prescription couldn't possibly have yielded.

As for those who warn of undescribed dangers of the biochemical-nutritional approach, don't be afraid to test the intellectual honesty of these prophets of an undefined doom. Just ask them for a description of the *known* side reactions which worry them. Also, and at the same time, request a list of the psychotropic drugs they dispense with so fine a "careless rapture," and *their known* side reactions.

It may be that your child has found the pathway to the normal and the real and the sane. In that happy case, you will need a knowledge of good nutrition to help keep him pointed in the right direction. But if he hasn't found it, he deserves a trial of the orthomolecular therapies—preferably through your own physician or psychiatrist, or from a specialist, if so it must be. My preference is for the cooperation of your own professional, for what he learns in the biochemical salvation of your child will be passed along to others.

·5·

Notes from an Orthomolecular Diary

A TASK FORCE for the American Psychiatric Association, assigned to an investigation of the claims made for orthomolecular treatment, condemned it on two prime grounds. No properly controlled research has been done, they said, which is blatantly untrue, and which implies that all the Ph.D.'s, and M.D.'s, biochemists, and psychiatrists who have conducted studies of orthomolecular and allied treatments are incompetent, which is both untrue and highly improbable. Second, the task force warned darkly that large doses of vitamins may somehow be dangerous, which indicates that they have chosen to ignore more than twenty years of skilled observations of thousands of patients—a majority, a *large* majority of whom have responded favorably to vitamin and collateral therapies, with no indication of any harm.

One envisions, from the A.P.A. task force reports, the orthomolecular practitioners as a group of self-deluded, wild-eyed, and scientifically incompetent fanatics, recklessly dosing helpless patients with medications not only useless but potentially harmful. Actually these men are at least as well trained as those who criticize them, and their studies far better controlled and more cautiously interpreted than many of those which are supposed to prove the value of psychoanalysis. In many cases the orthomolecular psychiatrists were initially unenthusiastic, but kept their minds open, and were certainly skeptical, but not cynical—a distinction which should be studied by another A.P.A. task force. One may logically ask what it was that persuaded talk-therapists, trained in and preoccupied with the dynamics of human personality, to immerse themselves in the alien field of cellular electron transport, vitamin-mineral-enzyme functions, impaired sugar tolerance, neuroallergy, and their roles in sicknesses of the human mind. A strong motivation is obvious: they were disillusioned with talk therapy as a treatment for schizophrenia, autism, and manic-depressive illnesses, for study after study confirmed their own experience: untreated patients had about the same recovery rate as those subjected to interminable hours on the couch or consultation chair, or in the group. Some of them realized that responses to tranquilizers, psychoenergizers and antidepressants, with all their (sometimes irreversible) side reactions, implied that the chemistry of the mind might well be a key to the riddle of mental sickness. Others were persuaded by their early ventures into orthomolecular treatment. A typical example of that process is related by a psychiatrist faced with the problems of a young mother of three children. She had been seriously ill mentally for about five years, during which time she had undergone, unsuccessfully, every treatment which the American Psychiatric Association finds meritorious, including shock therapy, insulin shock, tranquilizers, drugs, group and individual psychiatric treatment. Her physician had made an appointment for her with a neurosurgeon. She was to undergo a lobotomy, the ''ice-pick'' operation which often converts the mentally ill and violently disturbed patient into a mentally ill and undisturbed vegetable. Her family heard about megavitamin treatment, and asked the physician if he was willing to prescribe it. He indignantly refused, casting a determined vote for brain surgery rather than vitamin therapy. The family persisted. They withdrew the patient from the hospital and sent her to the psychiatrist, who was willing to try the new orthomolecular therapy. His skepticism vanished as, ten weeks later, she was normal. He remarked that one could talk to her at length, and never for a moment guess that she had ever been ill. The key to sanity for her was thyroid hormone, and goodly doses of vitamins I've discussed earlier. And how does the psychiatric establishment manage to dispose of thousands of patient histories like these? By calling the research uncontrolled, which is scientifically unjustified. The patient was the control. Her lack of response to all the orthodox treatments provided a baseline against which to plot her degree of response to the orthomolecular therapy. The establishment also warns that the response may be a placebo reaction, which is to say that the patient would have responded just as well if the vitamin capsules had been filled with an inert substance. To which the obvious reply is: where was the placebo effect when she was plied with drugs and tranquilizers, shocked electrically and with insulin, and made the target for hundreds of hours of psychiatric consultation, conversation, analysis and probing?

This book has been written as a guide for those who may profit by orthomolecular therapy, not as an attack on the older techniques. Since the establishment insists on playing the time-dishonored role of orthodoxy in obstructing progress, it might be useful here to remind the opposition of the glaring weakness of the type of therapy it espouses. Here, for instance, is the comment of a physician who, as a patient, was a participant in group therapy:

"We were encouraged to express our feelings about everything in general, including personal reactions with each other. Lord knows how many millions of words were spent, for such apparently small purpose. At times, the groups were sullen and uncommunicative. At other times, a patient would express or confess feelings of, let us say, anger, hatred, or lust. This apparently was what the psychiatrists wanted, but when the tears or the fuss had quieted down, there was no apparent result." He continued: "I know of two illegitimate children conceived during the 'treatment,' many broken marriages, and some suicides by discharged patients. These casualties might be considered as unhappy but necessary side effects of psychotherapy, but the lamentable truth is that the treatment was far from beneficial." He concluded: "I am convinced by bitter experience that psychotherapy is a doubtful and even dangerous tool.'' Precisely what the task force said about orthomolecular treatment!

What then is a schizophrenic, if not a casualty of stress, if not a product of too little or too much mother love, too rigid or too relaxed toilet training, an overindulgent or a preoccupied father, or an ill-timed leer in the eyes of schizoid parents? He is the unfortunate victim of an heredity which makes him use chemicals normal to the body in ways which are abnormal. These deranged processes result in the accumulation in the body of toxic substances which disturb the entire organism, for incalculable consequences may follow when alien molecules reach the brain and nervous system. Consider a familiar compound of molecules of carbon, oxygen, and hydrogen, readily ''burned'' by the body into harmless combustion products: carbon dioxide and water, which are easily eliminated by the organism. Could such a compound cause hallucinations? Delirium? Cerebral and mental deterioration? Ask the members of A.A., for the compound is alcohol.

Not only may the presence of alien molecules in the brain twist thought and distort emotion, but the *absence* of an adequate supply of requisite molecules may also create havoc. A missing nutrient interferes with the action of the enzyme which depends upon it, and the enzyme deficiency partially chokes the flame of life, forcing the brain to struggle to ''breathe'' in a cloud of the smoke of half-burned fuel. The chain of reactions in the chemistries of the brain, exquisitely sequenced, is detoured or partially blocked, exactly as the absence of but one worker on a conveyor-belt manufacturing line negates the activities of the workers whose functions follow and depend on his. So it is that deficiency of niacinamide in the diet at first subtly stifles the sense of humor, and later creates the psychosis of pellagra. A deficiency of riboflavin may cause significant mental depression. So will an inadequate intake of thiamin, which will also cause unusual belligerence and sensitivity to noise. Lack of pantothenic acid causes profound depression; so does deficiency in biotin, which is probably very rare. A lack of Vitamin B_{12} brings difficulties with concentration and memory, stuporous depression, and agitated, manic, and paranoid behavior. Insufficient intake of Vitamin B_6 may touch off convulsions in babies, and in the adult, depression, extreme nervousness, and confusion. This is one of the reasons for the melancholia some women experience when using birth-control pills, many of which contain a hormone that causes deficiency in Vitamin B_6. Gentle warning: don't dismiss vitamin deficiencies as the monopoly of the underprivileged. They occur on both sides of the railroad track. The fact that you can afford good food doesn't necessarily mean that you select it.

Conversely, added intake of some nutritional factors will sometimes improve the performance of brain and nervous system—not only in the psychotic, but in the "normal," too; not only in the retarded, but in the intelligent as well. The Russians use vitamin B_{15} in the treatment of the mentally retarded. Several American orthomolecular psychiatrists have commented on the action of this vitamin in improving speech in children; others find it valuable as an anti-allergy vitamin. Supplements of glutamic acid (a protein factor) or of glutamine, a related compound, have brought behavior improvement in elderly patients with psychiatric illness, and I have seen rises in the I.Q.'s of children given glutamic acid. They don't all respond, and responses differ in degree, nor does the protein factor convert an idiot into a genius; but occasionally nine or ten grams of glutamic acid (or a gram of glutamine) daily will produce impressive improvements in the ability to learn, to retain, and to recall. Supplements of tryptophane, another protein acid, have brought clinical improvement in schizophrenia, and have promoted more restful sleep in healthy individuals. Added intake of Vitamin C, in gram quantities and more, has been followed by improvement in depression and in paranoid symptom complexes. Administration of Vitamin B_6 by intramuscular injection has eliminated symptoms described as "neurasthenic." Supplements of riboflavin in some cases have reduced tremor and, in cases of compulsive eating, the vitamin has helped to reduce the tendency to nighttime raids on the refrigerator.

Removal of sugar from the diet, with necessary changes in the intakes of starch, protein, and fat to meet more precisely the needs and tolerances of the individual, have in both children and adults, reduced or eliminated anxiety, depression, claustrophobia; sexual impotence and frigidity in adults; and fatigability in all age groups. Such dietary changes have been very helpful in appropriate cases of schizophrenia, autism, and hyperactivity. Severe allergies, dyslexia, symptoms of brain damage, schizophrenia, autism, and learning difficulties in some children have responded to this type of diet.

The statements made in the preceding paragraphs are not only the author's educated opinions. They reflect the actual experiences of orthomolecular practitioners. One is driven to agree with Dr. Roger Williams when he remarks that if you escape mental disease, it isn't because you had shock treatment or the right tranquilizers, but because you have supplied all the minerals, amino acids, vitamins, and other factors your brain cells need to keep them in reasonably good working order.

However derived, the toxic chemicals which torture the nervous system and twist the perceptions of the schizophrenic convert his body and his world into the strange and the unreal. He perceives the changes but can't realize that they are based on aberrations of the chemistry of his own brain, and is convinced it is the external world which has altered. Thus nothing convinces a schizophrenic that the "voices" he hears originate within him, and are actually his own thoughts. You may in frustration show him textbooks in which auditory hallucinations are described as common in schizophrenia, and he will tell you that his case is the exception, and the voices *he* hears are real. To such dysperceptions he reacts in ways which to him (and to you, if you were in his place) seem appropriate, but obviously aren't to society. So begin consequences, not only for him, but for those who love him; for the broken mind, unlike the fractured bone, is infectious. We easily excuse the individual who can't run because he is on crutches. We can't adjust ourselves to the handicap of the "fractured" brain, for it poisons the relationships between the patient and those who cherish him, a situation in no way bettered by talk-therapists who "explain" the sickness as caused by the parents' sins of omission and commission, and fan the patient's hostilities until, sometimes tragically, they explode. There are better explanations, and they lead to better and more effective treatments. Newest of these, the ortho-molecular.

As an orthomolecular consultant to the profession, I have had a first-hand opportunity to watch as well as to institute and supervise such treatment programs. I have no vested interest in the field, though I confess freely to a strong bias in favor of the patient and his family and, for that reason, deeply regret and resent the obstructionist tactics of those who have a vested interest in older (and useless, and some-times harmful) techniques of treatment. For that reason, I should like to review some of the patient histories which molded my attitudes toward orthomolecular therapies and toward those who condemn them on a solid basis of no experience with them.

A San Francisco psychiatrist with whom I talked reviewed the history of many patients who have suffered from depres-sion or psychotic episodes, whose dietary histories proved later to be directly responsible for their troubles. He tells of a teacher who had been hospitalized for headaches, a sensa-tion of tightness in his chest, hyperventilation, racing pulse, muscle spasms, and general weakness. His attending physi-cian did not resort to the diagnosis which neatly (and un-helpfully) disposes of troublesome patients whose disorder escapes the practitioner's diagnostic skills: it's psychoso-matic. Instead he prescribed a hypoglycemia diet, which proved ineffective, but was nonetheless logical, for many pa-tients with low blood sugar have headaches, pulse irregular-ities, and muscle spasms. The psychiatrist, next to see the patient, was suspicious of a potassium deficiency, for it is capable of causing many of these symptoms. (You may recall that some of the astronauts suffered irregularities of the heart-beat, because of potassium deficiency, as the price for drinking synthetic instead of real orange juice.) A hair analysis for minerals showed potassium levels 50 percent below low-normal, and complete recovery followed a diet high in potassium-rich foods, with added supplements of the nutrient. At this point in this book, you should be ready to accept the concept, but before you read the first page, would you have believed that weakness, headache, pulse irregularities, and over-breathing could be successfully treated with bananas, tomato juice, orange juice, pecans, and raisins?

A neuroallergist was understandably proud of his success in rescuing a teenager who had been repeatedly hospitalized as psychotic because of her suicidal depression, which nothing in her life situation justified. Three years of hospitalization, with repeated bouts of shock therapy and a long list of psychoenergizing drugs brought her even farther from reality. Tests for allergy produced dizziness and anxiety; the chlorine in drinking water turned on her suicidal depression; eating lamb caused confusion and anxiety. She is well now, and stays that way by avoiding the allergens that wracked her mind.

Another allergist tested a young man who was complaining of severe fatigue, mental confusion, and nervous tension. A talk-therapist had assured the patient that emotional stress was the basic cause of his troubles, but in no less than fifteen tests, his reactions to common foods reproduced all his "emotional" symptoms, including those which had made him a source of an annuity for a psychoanalyst. When he learned to avoid milk, coffee, chicken, eggs, peas, corn, and other foods to which he was sensitive, his "emotional" troubles evaporated.

With a diagnosis of a severe mental breakdown, a middle-aged housewife became a patient in a psychiatric hospital, where it was apparent that she suffered with hallucinations and delusions. Vitamin B_{12}, given by intramuscular injection, ended her illness. The response to this treatment was the same in an eighty-four-year-old woman, diagnosed as a "senile dement'' and confined in a geriatric ward in a large hospital. Her physician gave her injections of Vitamin B_{12} and its co-worker, folic acid. Her response was, her physician remarked, ''an unexpectedly rapid return to intellectual and behavioral normality.'' He added that it was interesting that she could not remember anything of the period when she was psychotic. Two points of great interest are reflected in these cases treated with Vitamin B_{12}: contrary to what physicians were taught just a decade ago, the vitamin was specifically helpful even though no sign of pernicious anemia, for which Vitamin B_{12} is ordinarily used, existed. Second: there are still medical ''authorities'' who tell their colleagues that the only excuse for using Vitamin B_{12} therapeutically *is* pernicious anemia. Obstructionism is not confined to psychiatrists of an outmoded philosophy.

I asked an orthomolecular psychiatrist why he had discarded his couch in favor of foods and vitamins. He remarked that he used to ''treat'' schizophrenia by psychoanalysis, digging into the mind to bring up subconscious material. It was a comfortable practice which had only one drawback: the patients didn't get better. He became frustrated with the non-productive talk-tranquilizer treatment, turned to megavitamin therapy, and found his patients were not only getting well, but contrary to all experience with all therapies for schizophrenics, were *staying* well. Other physicians, he noted, were fascinated with his results, and adopted the new approach. Blanket resistance came from psychiatrists, primarily, who obviously were condemning the treatment without having observed it. One of his patients was the clinical psychologist who, with his help, struggled from the depths of catatonic schizophrenia, and whose story is told in Chapter One. She is back in practice.

Although vitamin therapy dominated the orthomolecular scene for many years, the work of Pfeiffer and other pioneers has now placed equal emphasis on minerals. A psychiatrist reviews the story of a young woman who complained of severe depression, sudden losses of energy that prevented her from accomplishing necessary, everyday household chores, and occasional but frightening impulses toward suicide, unexplained by her life situation but increasingly difficult to combat. Tests of her hair showed a deficiency in copper, but her diet seemed adequately supplied with the metal, which implied a difficulty in absorption or utilization. The physician gave her chelated copper, a form which is efficiently absorbed. A week later she reported that she had resumed menstruating, cessation of which had depressed her because she was persuaded that she was going into very premature menopause. This for her was tantamount to premature aging. With the psychological stress and the copper deficiency removed, she was quickly back to normal.

Lithium has been found useful as an antidepressant, which is interesting because lithiated mineral waters have been used from time immemorial for "nervous disorders." A distinguished psychiatrist reports on four schizophrenics who received "significant help from adding lithium carbonate" to their intake of megavitamins and/or tranquilizers. The first patient was a young man who at nineteen was a seven-year veteran of hospitalization for schizophrenia. He came to the psychiatrist from a state institution, where it was reported that he had been allowed to leave the hospital for a few weekend visits to his home, but he always returned in a regressed and disorganized state which necessitated increased tranquilization. The hospital staff blamed his mother's dominating attitude for the patient's relapse. His psychiatric testing showed a high score for paranoid symptoms and for distortions of perception. His moods were erratic and unpredictable. Watching football games on TV, he became hyperactive and disorganized, so excited that he was out of control, no matter to what heights the psychiatrist raised the tranquilizer doses. He was given large amounts of niacin and Vitamin C, plus electric shock treatment, but the acutely disturbed episodes still occurred. Now the psychiatrist added lithium to the prescription. The young man, who had never been able to hold a job before, obtained his first position. He completed two years of college, and held several part-time positions to help pay his expenses. There has been no evidence of psychosis or neurosis, and no episodes of acute disturbance. The vitamin prescription, the tranquilizer—in very small doses—and the lithium have been continued.*

Another patient was a forty-one-year-old woman who was first hospitalized for marked mental deterioration in 1965. Her illness began after the birth of her only child, which brought her into psychotherapy for fourteen years. Despite the treatment, she became an alcoholic, and was heavily medicated with four tranquilizers (simultanously), though without benefit. The orthomolecular psychiatrist remarks that although she had never been hospitalized before, she had the appearance of a chronic hospital patient, which is, if you have seen it, unforgettable—her face expressionless and fixed, her answers to questions halting and indecisive. She reflected an atmosphere of fear, hopelessness, and, at times, suspiciousness. Sporadic blocking of her speech suggested a catatonic state. Electroshock treatments brought some improvement in that she was more sociable but lacked self-confidence. Her compulsive use of alcohol persisted, and was treated with Antabuse. The orthomolecular psychiatrist prescribed niacin, ascorbic acid, and a thyroid supplement, and there was a gradual improvement in her interests and activities. She had several setbacks, after the last of which she was deeply depressed, with psychomotor retardation that didn't respond to medication. Accordingly, the psychiatrist gave her lithium carbonate. Two weeks of this therapy, and she felt normal. She is now a part-time teacher's assistant in an elementary school and works part-time in her husband's professional office, while finding time and psychic energy to care for her aging and ailing parents. She appears, the psychiatrist notes, to be living a relatively normal life, "which is more than was ever expected by anyone, including the patient." The psychiatrist interprets his results with the statement that when the schizophrenic features of the illness are controlled

---

*A new form of lithium—lithium orotate—has been introduced. This permits dosage to be very much smaller than that required for the carbonate.

with megavitamins and/or tranquilizers, the manic-depressive features become more obvious and can be properly treated.

Why all the excitement about lithium, when there are dozens of antidepressant drugs available? For the simple reason that lithium manages to restrain the flight of the psychic pendulum without stifling the patient's creativity. The drugs tend to smother it.

The Russian use of Vitamin B_{15} (pangamic acid), a nutrient not recognized by the F.D.A. (which makes it no less valuable), has been mentioned. Stocks in the United States are slender and virtually constitute a black market, which has, of course, impeded research with this factor, despite the fact that it was first recognized and concentrated by an American biochemist. One psychiatrist believes it to be an important part of the treatment of speech development, and very useful in helping the allergic. He tells the story of a little boy who was hyperactive, had temper tantrums, couldn't be toilet trained, and spoke such a garbled language that not a word could be understood. Megavitamin therapy with niacin, Vitamin C, and Vitamin B_6 produced no response. The orthomolecular practitioner decided as a last resort to try the effect of Vitamin B_{15}, in doses of 300 mgs. a day. It was speculative therapy, not because it is dangerous, but because the prior principal use for the vitamin, largely in Europe, had been in the treatment of disorders of the heart and the blood vessels. After a month of Vitamin B_{15} therapy, his mother brought the boy back to the psychiatrist, who noted that the youngster was sitting quietly in his chair, with none of the usual uproar. He asked the mother about her observations of the young patient. In answer, she said: "Johnnie, count." The child counted up to fifteen. She gratefully told the doctor that the boy was toilet trained, and that his speech had developed unbelievably within the one month.

Apropos of the imputed failure of orthomolecular psychiatrists to perform controlled research, one of the pioneers in this field has had the rare opportunity to study identical twins, eleven pairs, all schizophrenic. In every instance, he points out, the twin treated with diet and vitamins has recovered or is recovering. In every instance, the "control" twin is still sick and is not recovering. He cites the story of identical twin girls, suffering from recurrent attacks of schizophrenia for twenty-five years. One of them happened to visit a medical nutritionist, complaining of back pain; he diagnosed the schizophrenia, and treated it with a supervised diet and megavitamins. She has been more or less well for the past four or five years, with one or two minor relapses. The other twin, being treated with drugs and tranquilizers by psychiatrists hostile to the orthomolecular approach, has been in mental hospitals twelve times during the same period.

There are twilight zone psychoses, sometimes called "borderline schizophrenia." A patient so diagnosed, with strong paranoid tendencies, was a twenty-four-year-old unmarried woman who had spent ten years in psychotherapy, with three different therapists. She never progressed beyond that "borderline" classification, but her paranoia prevented her from holding a job or a boyfriend, or making close friends. The usual psychotropic drugs were unhelpful, and had unpleasant side effects. Her therapist finally placed her on a sugar-free diet, with no explanation, except that it might help her to take off weight. He adopted this approach because her unfortunate experiences with medication had made her suspicious of all such therapeutic procedures. For that reason, when she was given megavitamin treatment, the only explanation was that the vitamins might give her more energy, a possibility she grasped because she suffered from apathy and listlessness. Within a few months she demonstrated a different emotional tone, in which she discarded the hostile and paranoid element in her interactions with others. For the first time in her life she made a friend and, subsequently, she acquired and maintained a continuing relationship with a boyfriend. Previously she had been so hypercritical that young men seldom called her for a second date. She was also newly able to hold a position, and to get along with her superiors. This contrasted sharply with the past, when she had always become paranoid, and had been discharged or quit her position indignantly because of fancied wrongs. She subsequently married, had two children, and is functioning normally as a housewife. Because the stress of childbirth often causes flaring of psychosis, her vitamin intake was increased temporarily after the birth of each child.

A forty-one-year-old housewife had been hospitalized fifteen times in seven years for acute schizophrenic episodes which could not be controlled with drugs, in whatever amount and type they were prescribed. The attacks were always preceded by a period of difficulty in sleeping, and often occurred during the premenstrual week. Between attacks, her psychometric tests showed her to be virtually normal. In addition to a hypoglycemia diet and megavitamins, she was given a sizable dose of thyroid, a hormone treatment suggested by the association between her menstrual cycle and the schizophrenic episodes. Since that prescription, she has not had a single recurrence. She functions and feels as though she had never been ill.

A fascinating example of distortion of perception occurred in a teacher, working toward her master's degree, who had gradually changed from a pleasant and well-liked person to one moody, withdrawn, and depressed. She was fully conscious of the ways in which she perceived changes in the world around her, particularly because friends who had taken psychedelic drugs told her that their experiences were similar. As an example, she could see the pattern of a rug hovering in the air about twelve inches above the carpet itself and appearing, while suspended in midair, to ripple, she said, in a pleasing way. She wondered if she was developing schizophrenia, which had been described to her as "tripping—without taking LSD." Her score on a test for schizophrenia was very high, indicating widespread and severe disorganization of her perceptions of reality. The orthomolecular psychiatrist explained her illness to her as a chemical disturbance of the brain and prescribed megavitamins, a hypoglycemic diet, and low dosages of tranquilizers. She was then retested monthly. Her high score for schizophrenia gradually and steadily dropped, and as it did, her symptoms in like proportion diminished. This doesn't always happen; sometimes the test scores show a significant improvement before the behavior and the dysperceptions change enough for the therapist to be aware of the progress. Seven months after the start of treatment, her elevated schizophrenia score had been reduced by almost 88 percent. At this point she felt that she needed some psychotherapy, to deal with emotional problems she wanted to discuss. Which is fine; but what would the prognosis have been if psychotherapy alone had been employed from the start of her illness? Would the rippling image above the carpet have returned to its proper place?

When hypoglycemia complicates and aggravates schizophrenic symptoms, as it does in more than half the cases, control of the diet becomes a basic part of the treatment. This is emphasized in the history of a male schizophrenic who had been ill for several years, hospitalized several times, and treated with electric shock and all other available forms of therapy. He was described as surly, uncooperative, paranoid, and obese. A glucose tolerance test revealed hypoglycemia, and he was placed on the usual regimen of megavitamins, a tranquilizer, and a caffeine-and-sugar-free diet—with absolutely no progress for the next one and one-half years. His family then discovered that he was drinking at least half a case of cola beverage daily during the week, and doubling that intake on the weekend. When this was stopped, there was rapid, progressive improvement in his behavior, his ability to communicate, and his relationship with his family. His inappropriate responses and his surly, crude manner disappeared, and he is continuing to improve.

The persistance of the patient, in the preceding history, in consuming large amounts of a beverage saturated with sugar and high in caffeine, a procedure calculated to make his condition worse, is characteristic of some schizophrenics, who manage to negate every effort to help them, as if the disease were a shield they are unwilling to drop. There is always the possibility that the patient is addicted to the foods and beverages to which he is sensitive or allergic. In a hypoglycemic, the initial effect of caffeine and sugar is a stimulation. The price paid for it is depression, irritability, weakness, and worsening of the symptoms of psychosis; but the advent of these disturbances is frequently the opportunity for the patient, seeking restimulation, to resume his intake of the offending food or beverage, and so is the vicious cycle perpetuated. Occasionally the patient is not a voluntary victim of the bad habit, but his peers or his parents become advocates. I recall a New York psychiatrist who could not persuade the patient's mother that her son, who had largely been normalized by a hypoglycemia diet and megavitamins, was literally being pressed into psychotic behavior by the cola drinks, candy, and cookies with which she "rewarded" him. The psychiatrist, in her presence, gave the twenty-six-year-old several bottles of a cola drink; half an hour later the patient was lying on the floor, weeping, curled up in the fetal position with his thumb in his mouth, and calling for his mother—who was within arm's reach of him. "Oh, my God!" she murmured. "I didn't realize . . ." She might be echoed by the talk-therapist who tries to treat such a patient by probing his subconscious.

Bypassing the patient's resistance to treatment sometimes draws upon the ingenuity of both the family and the practitioner. A forty-four-year-old man was a veteran of ten years of chronic paranoid schizophrenia. He had been given up as hopeless after many years of conventional treatment. His family protected him, as best they could, by keeping him at home, in his own room, but his behavior was so disturbed that the situation became unbearable. He shouted obscenities at imaginary enemies, refused to change clothes or take medication, and showed no interest in external events. The family heard of orthomolecular treatment and took him to a clinic where, with the help of the psychiatrist, they developed a combination of vitamins combined with enough bicarbonate of soda to neutralize the acidity of the niacin, plus chicory for flavoring. This was then surreptitiously added to everything he drank. After a few months, he began to respond and improve, and the psychiatrist hastened the process by adding a liquid tranquilizer to the formula. A year later, he was voluntarily well-dressed, no longer hallucinated, carried on normal conversations, read the papers, watched television (which, cynically, might have been a residual psychotic symptom) and was well on his way to mental health. Two years later, he was planning to live on his own, which confronted the family with a problem, since he was unaware that he had been given the covert vitamin treatment. They decided to act as if this were a new suggestion, and recommended that he take the vitamin formula, which he rejected. After all, he reminded them, he had been doing pretty well on his own for the last few years!

It was perhaps five years ago that a research psychiatrist invited me to test nutritional therapies on patients in one of New York State's giant mental hospitals. I refused when I learned that my cases would be a "back ward" group—chronic schizophrenics, so long hospitalized and so sick that organic brain damage must have occurred, so that nothing short of biological dynamite would stir them. I may have been wrong in that refusal. Consider the history of a thirty-year-old schizophrenic who had been under treatment for fifteen years, with six hospitalizations, a full course of insulin shock, and over one-hundred electric shock treatments. Her family, understandably, was ready to give up and place her in a state institution, for she was incontinent, wouldn't wear her false teeth, constantly rocked, and would not communicate with her parents. She was treated with a hypoglycemia diet, megavitamins, tranquilizers, and thyroid. There was a very slow and partial response; yet at the two-year mark, her appearance was much improved, she wore her teeth and used makeup, spoke politely, and had achieved bowel and bladder control. The family no longer felt distressed in traveling in public with her, or in having her participate in family social visits. Her emotional tone was still flat, her behavior still moderately strange, and her overall style was still stilted and somewhat awkward, but you can understand that her family gratefully accepted her limited progress.

In the course of treating patients with vitamins and diet, the practitioner often is reminded that schizophrenia is a physical disease. A pioneering psychiatrist in this field interviewed a chronic schizophrenic, a woman who had, according to her husband, responded sharply to orthomolecular treatment. Both the patient and her husband urged the doctor to examine her nails, on which appeared a graphic reflection of her "mental" illness. The forward half of the nail was yellow-brown; the half toward the cutical, a normal pink. The line between the two was sharp, and appeared in the same relative position in each nail. It became apparent that a few months earlier she had stopped depositing schizophrenic pigment in her nails—probably quite suddenly, since the margin between the two areas was so sharp. This observation was echoed by another patient of the same practitioner, who reported that while she was sick, her nails didn't grow and required no cutting. After a week of the megavitamin therapy, they began to grow normally, and were pinker—transmitting light better—than before. The reader should be reminded of the white spots in the nails, reported as part of the Sara syndrome, in Chapter Three.

As treatment for low blood sugar has been used to help both schizophrenics and alcoholics, so have large doses of niacinamide helped both groups. A specialist in alcoholism observes that the vitamin shows marked ability to reduce the mood swings and insomnia common in alcoholics. It helps to stabilize behavior so that other treatments for alcoholism become more efficient, and it reduces or changes the effect of alcohol on the individual, drinking becoming less rewarding when niacinamide is used. The vitamin also lessens the severity of withdrawal symptoms. It is not a cure for the alcoholic, but an important addition to the traditional treatment. Alcoholism has largely been dominated by talk-therapy. The disorder is described as an escape from reality, which begs the question: why not blondes, the stock market, TV, or bowling? Why such a self-punishing "escape"? In an earlier book, I presented a small but, I believe, convincing amount of evidence to indicate that *some* alcoholics are the victims of hypoglycemia at first, and alcoholism second, as a perverted expression of the disturbance in carbohydrate metabolism. In these cases, treatment of the underlying condition—low blood sugar—wipes out the drinking. By that statement, I mean that such an alcoholic, without vows, promises, or religious revelations, will stop drinking; should he choose to drink, he stops when he chooses. But the establishment in alcoholism is like that in psychiatry, which is not coincidence when psychiatric theory has been the only peg on which treatment for alcoholism has hung its therapeutic hat, and this patent fact is ignored: the alcoholic population isn't homogeneous. We should not talk of "the brain" as if there were only one model; of "brain chemistry" as if there were but one kind; nor of "the alcoholic," for the same reason.

A psychiatrist—*not* orthomolecular—in a letter to a major medical journal, reported both success and failure in his testing of the megavitamin therapy. One of his cases responded in a way which elicited from him a stern statement to his colleagues. In malignant conditions like schizrenia, he observed, the physician is ethically obliged to use first any or all of the "accepted" therapies. If these fail to produce an optimum response, he must add any safe medication that conceivably might help the patient. The case which spurred him into writing the declaration was that of a twenty-five-year-old catatonic schizophrenic, restless, disturbed, and noisy. Electric shock treatment produced temporary improvement, with rapid relapse. Insulin shock had the same aftermath. She was emotionally very flat, with a vacant and apathetic face. She was preoccupied, with severe thought disorder and blocking of thoughts, and she had auditory hallucinations of people calling her name. In eight days of doses of five grams of niacinamide daily, she showed more initiative, and said she felt better. She was still apathetic, but she smiled spontaneously, and reported her hallucinations were gone. Five days later she was speaking quite naturally, had lost her vacant look, and was obviously much improved. Twenty-one days later she was taking care of her personal appearance, going into town, visiting with her friends, and no longer getting lost. Her thinking seemed almost normal, although she retained an odd difficulty in comprehending proverbs. She was discharged, subsequently married, and had three children. There was a relapse after the birth of her third child—childbirth often presents this hazard—but she responded fully to tranquilizers, and has remained well and free of symptoms. The psychiatrist cautiously admits that the result might be due to chance, but points out that she had shown no improvement whatsoever prior to taking niacinamide, and that the type of schizophrenia she had (hebrephrenia) is one which rarely has spontaneous recoveries. If orthomolecular treatment helps but one such patient in twenty, who has the right to make it difficult for the patient to receive the therapy?

A long perspective on groups of psychotics answers that question more explicit than do individual patient histories. There were two groups of schizophrenics treated at a Canadian hospital between 1955 and 1962. Seventy-six received megavitamin therapy, and 226 were treated in the older ways. During the 7 years, 21 patients on vitamin therapy were readmitted to the hospital for a total of 43 times, spending 2,453 days in the institution. Four are now in it. None committed suicide. In the larger group, given the older therapies, 122 were readmitted to the hospital 275 times, for a total stay of more than 25,000 days. Seventeen of these are still hospitalized; 4 killed themselves. A little mental arithmetic demonstrates that on orthomolecular treatment, a higher percentage of patients recover and remain well; a smaller percentage has to return to the hospital, and their stays are shorter, and there is a significant difference in the suicidal tendency so characteristic of schizophrenics. The Task Force negative report notwithstanding, the biochemical type of treatment obviously restores to society many useful individuals whose chances of getting lost in the byways of Freudian double-talk would otherwise, unfortunately, be excellent.

With the drama of responses to orthomolecular treatment of the psychotic and the neurotic, we may forget how heartwarming it is to use nutrition to improve mental function in college or high school drop-outs, or to restore normal thinking in the aged where time itself (senility) is being blamed for what is actually the price of long-term malnutrition. "Swimmy-headedness" or mental confusion is one of the preludes to outright pellagra, but it also appears—and yields to nutritional treatment—in individuals who never develop pellagra. This is to say that the "metabolic dysperception" described in children who respond to doses of niacinamide has its counterpart in adults who are in touch with reality, but see it through clouded glasses.

By the same token, teachers are learning that lethargic, inattentive children, as well as some of those who are disruptive in the classroom, are often those who come to school without breakfast. "Nervous" children, described as well-nourished by average medical standards, often improve when deprived of cola beverages and candy, and with the addition to their menus of a midmorning, high-protein snack, which may be nothing more esoteric than a glass of milk.

Since time is a measure of duration, and nothing more, "senility" is a tag, not an explanation, for the agitated and confused behavior of aged individuals. I personally have often seen, and the medical literature has repeatedly reported, improvements in alertness, concentration and memory spans, and clarity of thinking in the elderly, merely by improvement of the diet and proper use of supplements of the Vitamin B complex, Vitamin C, trace minerals, and Vitamin E. While the establishment scoffs at the use of food concentrates, it can do so only by ignoring pertinent findings by objective scientific groups—the geriatric division of the National Institutes of Health, for instance, who found one-third of a group of *affluent* senior citizens to be deficient in Vitamin B complex.

Similarly, the emphasis on low blood sugar as part of the problems of the autistic, withdrawn, and schizophrenic children, as well as those with dyslexia, hyperactivity, and learning difficulties, and the references to hypoglycemia as a complication of the troubles of the schizophrenic should not be allowed to obscure the fact that this disorder will cause symptoms of psychosis in mentally *normal* individuals, will simulate neurosis in individuals who are *not* neurotic, and can lower the level of physical and mental functioning of those who have been assured that they are in perfect health. One of my colleagues, a specialist in hypoglycemia, is a neuropsychiatrist in Ohio who has published a list of the erroneous diagnoses made on patients who actually were suffering from nothing more than low blood sugar. Thirty-eight were told they had ''psychoneurotic depression.'' Thirty-three were said to be suffering from ''depressive reaction.'' Six had been told they were paranoid schizophrenics, four were labeled ''undifferentiated schizophrenics,'' two were tagged with ''schizo-affective psychosis,'' another four were accused of ''maniac-depressive psychosis,'' two women were informed that their trouble was postpartum depression, three cases were grouped as ''psychopathic personality,'' three were supposed to be victims of marital maladjustment, and nine cases were classified as chronic alcoholism—which it was, but it was based on hypoglycemia, and disappeared when the low blood sugar was treated.

These, obviously, though not psychotic or severely neurotic individuals, were seriously disturbed by hypoglycemia. The disorder may have more subtle effects, never severe enough to bring the individual to a psychiatrist. A feeling of depersonalization—of being two individuals in one body, coupled with a sense of detachment from reality; belligerence abnormal to the usual personality; recurrent and unexplained anxiety—these and a half-hundred other impediments to social and vocational functioning are among the penalties for low blood sugar. The following is one of literally a hundred thousand letters which reached me from readers of my book on hypoglycemia:

Without getting into too much detail, my father went through two years of sheer hell simply because he was suffering from undetected hypoglycemia. It was not until I came across your book in the local library that I realized that most of his symptoms matched the ones outlined in your book. As you predicted, it was most difficult for our family to obtain a sugar-tolerance test for him; our doctor, whom, incidentally, we have dropped, preferred to think of my father as a hypochondriac, neurotic, and alcoholic. Finally, my family literally demanded that the test be given. As it turned out, my father suffers from severe hypoglycemia, but since following your diet, plus a few tips begrudgingly given by the doctor, he is today a new man.

What fortified the physician's resistance? The attitude of the A.M.A. toward hypoglycemia? Or, if he was a psychiatrist, the philosophy of the Task Force on Orthomolecular Psychiatry? Even within the ranks of these establishment fortresses, there are dissenters—and the truth will, as it always does, one day find its way up to the hierarchy. My good friend, Dr. E. Cheraskin, points out that psychiatrists *usually* conduct no physical examinations, and those who fail to discover brain tumors and glandular disturbances are unlikely to uncover elusive conditions like magnesium deficiency, hypoglycemia, or dysperception metabolically based on niacin dependency. He quotes an official of the American Psychiatric Association as remarking that the failure of psychiatrists to pay heed to physical disorders borders on malpractice, and as making the prophecy that eventually when the psychiatric profession will have buried itself in its psychoanalytic theories, the profession will then be taken over by scientists who understand biochemistry and metabolic medicine. The process will take, he estimates, twenty-five years.

That's too long a cultural lag, even in medicine, notorious for such gaps. And that is why this book was written. If it rescues one child from schizophrenia, if it returns one dropout to college, if it saves *one* person in a hundred from sitting in the gray day-room of a mental institution, vegetating under the impact of the latest tranquilizer, it will have served its purpose.

How well it may serve that purpose is graphically illustrated in the letter which follows. It is not only a record of a heartwarming triumph of orthomolecular treatment of a child schizophrenic, but it is also a monument to the therapeutic opportunities which remain unrecognized in the conventional psychiatric approaches to the problem.

Dear Doctor————:

Mary and I watched the Merv Griffin show last week, and heard Dr. Carlton Fredericks tell the whole country the story of Sara and 110 others like her; and we assume and hope Mary is included in these fantastic statistics.

This is really a cover letter for Mary's history, which you requested some time ago. First, though, let me tell you about her today. She has energy to spare. All the mysterious aches and pains have almost disappeared. She had the flu only once this winter. Three of her stories have been entered into the National Scholastic Achievement Award contest and we know she is among the finalists. Her grades are A's (with an A in phys. ed. based on "sportsmanship," indicating her relationship to others). Mary is also singing solos in her school's spring concert, and has a lead in the school play. She has a hobby for the first time, old movies, and her attention span allows her now to enjoy watching them. The most amazing thing is her ability to handle a busy schedule efficiently. Anyone who has not seen Mary for a period of time is dramatically impressed with our new girl. Those who see her daily are also very aware of the change.

I must explain that Mary has always been a good student, has strived for a good relationship with her family and friends; and appeared "normal" for the most part to the world; however, we all know now the stress she was functioning under. Our physicians, while good men, still seem reluctant to accept this cure; but gradually they seem to be accepting the obvious.

(Note the last sentence: physicians not only balk at the concept of the orthomolecular approach to mental disease—they are reluctant to accept the cures!)

Mary's mother than appends the history of this "schizophrenic" child, actually suffering from a version of the Sara syndrome:

Mary spent her first three months [of life] screaming because of the colic. When she was approximately four years old, she went through a period of extreme exhaustion, would become quite pale and need bed rest. All kinds of tests were done, with no conclusive results. One pediatrician told us it was the way we were handling her. We changed doctors; the next man thought it truly physical in origin, and yet could find nothing wrong.

New situations always seemed traumatic for her and caused great anxiety. She was especially susceptible to infections, viruses, etc.

At age seven, she again suffered from extreme exhaustion following a bout with a sore throat. [Note the poor resistance of these schizophrenics to stress, explaining Dr. Pfeiffer's description of the Sara syndrome as a stress-induced psychosis.] She seemed to be having trouble adjusting to the new school situation and relating to other children, although her school work was fine and she did have neighborhood friends. Again, she had many tests; the only possibility raised was that she might have had infectious mononucleosis. Once more we changed doctors, but there were no specific problems or test results during the next year or so, except for a weight gain and eye problems requiring glasses.

We moved to another area, and Mary started school, but reacted to the new situation by becoming ill, exhausted, and having knee problems and chest pains. She had bumped her knee, just before we moved. She was hospitalized this time, tested for arthritis, mono, hearing problems; she was X-rayed from head to toe, checked for diabetes, kidneys, etc. Once more the only possibility was perhaps mono. She was out of school for six months, saw three orthopedic specialists, had one leg in a cast for six weeks, was told by another she was a hypochondriac or "pretending." Another orthopedist could see nothing wrong, and prescribed the cast for "general treatment and rest." The third could see and show us the obvious physical appearance of her bad knee as similar to a "football knee."

She spent the year suffering from various aches and pains, having trouble relating to the new school situations and some children here. Let me say that this problem was real, and other new students had difficulty being accepted, but the problem for Mary was handling the situation.

The following year she again experienced the total exhaustion she suffered previously, was once more hospitalized, once more had the battery of tests. This time, they were more complicated because she had a slight case of hepatitis. She was out of school again for weeks with exhaustion, chest pains, knee pains, nausea, etc., caused by the hepatitis. During this time she was checked for allergies, with no positive results. The chest pains grew worse, the abdominal pains increased, she seemed extra nervous, her attention span grew short, she had difficult in sleeping, and was especially sensitive to viruses and sore throats. Her knees bothered her to the point where we had to discontinue dancing and sometimes phys. ed. The doctor thought it was a problem common at her age.

She was tense and several times felt that people and children were talking about her, and being physically cruel and critical; I guess she was feeling persecuted. Again, let me stress that other children here had problems as newcomers or if they were exceptional children. Mary had her situation magnified by her inability to handle it.

We changed physicians, from the pediatrician to our family doctor. With him, we decided a tonsillectomy might help solve some of the throat, ear, and cold problems. Apparently it did, as this is no longer a difficulty. She still had pains around her spleen, and severe abdominal pains. Once we took her to the emergency room, and she was also checked by my gynecologist. Around this time, she had her first period and then no more. It was discovered that her eosinophil count was twenty-five percent when she had her tonsillectomy, and considering all her symptoms our doctor wanted to hospitalize her once more and check for trichinosis. Oh, yes, I almost forgot: two other big problems that went on for a long time—her eyes were constantly swollen, and her muscles ached.

Mary refused to go to the hospital again, and came home from school with some information that had been given her about a doctor who had treated another girl in our community, and the dramatic results. Obviously, doctor, the rest is in your file. We admit to being skeptical when told her blood chemistry would be normal in one week, and so waited two weeks to have it checked. It was normal, and so is Mary. No more aches and pains, no exhaustion, her periods are regular, etc.

Because of our experience with preconceived ideas regarding these problems, and with the label "schizophrenic," we have asked our family physician not to enter Mary's psychological test results in her medical file here. He has seen all the laboratory results conducted at your facility, and everything else is on record. If you should decide to use Mary as a case history, please use only her first name, as you did with Sara. Mary's attitude is changing, and she now is beginning to be proud of the good results instead of self-conscious about them, but we respect her desire that the psychological test results not follow her, unless by her choice. Thank you for our daughter . . .
Sincerely,

Thank you for our daughter. She might have written "Thank you for being the kind of psychiatrist-biochemist who, viewing the psychiatric disorders without a closed mind, with a 'child's unbiased eye,' was perfectly willing to drop the sterile and traditional approaches, and to explore—so fruitfully—the uses of the molecules of sanity."

· 6 ·

The Flame of Sanity

THERE IS A genetic disease of children marked by compulsive chewing of their lips and fingers, which continues until they are heartbreakingly mutilated. That symptom and the mental retardation accompanying it are the result of a disturbance of adrenal function and of an enzyme chemistry, nothing more, and the disorder is an example of a psychochemical disease— a tragic reminder that molecules mold the mind. For the brain and nervous system are exquisitely sensitive to disturbances of body chemistry which may not noticeably affect other organs. A chronic defect in the utilization of sugar in the body may not cause a single physical symptom, though it often does—but it can make you claustrophobic or a hypochondriac, fill you with obsessive and unbased fears, or prod you into alcoholism or asthma. Elevation of the lactic acid in your blood will not ravage the body, but it can inflict on you a constant sense of impending doom, which isn't made more tolerable by the fact that you know of no valid reason for the feeling. Even so apparently minor a factor as inadequate oxidation (burning) of starches and sugars in the body may cause you to feel alienated from and distrustful of others, even those to whom you are emotionally close. If your dietary scale is tipped in the direction of too much starch and sugar, you may wind up, as one young woman did, afraid of everything, from large glass windows (they might break) to bridges (they might fall) to elevators (they might drop).

With the complexities of the external and internal environments in which we try to maintain a dynamic balance, it takes only a few wrong molecules to twist, to disarray, or even to interrupt the intricately linked sequences of the chemistries of the brain. (At this moment, some of your brain cells are dying, as they do every minute in every one of us. Some of them die prematurely from lack of Vitamin E, needed to protect them against cosmic irradiation. This is true of all human cells.) Inadequate nutrition, obviously, is a frequent factor in causing chemical chaos in the body, with inevitable repercussions on mind and personality, sometimes unaccompanied by *physical* signs of nutritional deficiency disease. The vitamin deficiency that causes shortening of the concentration and memory spans need not be severe enough to give you neuritis; that which makes you irritable and dampens your sense of humor is usually far too mild to cause pellagra. An unbalanced diet can make you hear voices that are not there, or cause you to feel like two people in one body, one watching the other—and the worst part of having such symptoms is the fact that no physician or psychiatrist, unless trained in the orthomolecular approach, will be persuaded that such symptoms can coexist with sanity. If you eat too much sugar, an indirect result can be insomnia of a type which awakens you at two in the morning and will not let you return to sleep; or it can cause terrifying nightmares, which leave you dripping with perspiration, and with a feeling that a band is tightening across your chest and interfering with your breathing. A diet low in fat, though for opposite biochemical reasons, may cause the same symptoms—and with them, what are your chances of winding up on a psychiatric couch, reviewing your childhood toilet training for a noncommital psychoanalyst?

Though a diet high in the type of protein called "purines" threatened some people with gout, lack of enough of such foods—liver, other organ meats, yeast, asparagus, and others—may in some people create a restricted potential in mental, emotional, and physical functioning. If your body burns sugar too quickly, you may develop most of the symptoms

return. She then started a low carbohydrate reducing diet. This was the prelude to her attacks of melancholia, and it became easy therefore to trace the chemical upset that touched them off. She had depressed the bacterial flora (those normal to the lower bowel) by use of the drug. The bacteria would probably have regrown when the medication was stopped, but the low carbohydrate diet deprived them of the constituent of food they critically need for growth. The combined insult upset the nutrition of the body, and the impact showed in moodiness and depression, both vanishing when she increased her intake of starch and reimplanted friendly bacteria by the generous daily use of yogurt.*

Physical disturbances and diseases have long been blamed on factors of stress and depletion, but it is a comparatively recent realization that they can cause a wide spectrum of psychiatric symptoms, ranging all the way from simple moodiness to extreme abnormality—including psychosis. These symptoms may include such "personality traits" as lack of confidence, apathy, and shyness, and such "emotional" and "mental" disorders as disturbances of perception in hearing, touch, and vision; paranoid feelings of distrust and suspicion; vague fears, anger, irritability, sadness, and introversion of a normally outgoing personality. These all become puzzling and doubly disturbing when they are alien to the individual's accustomed behavior, can't be explained by the life situation or blamed on his mother, and can't be controlled.

The search for such physical entities in diseases classically considered purely mental is not only pressingly urgent (even if palpably rejected by psychiatrists): it is mandatory. Almost a century ago, a psychiatrist pertinently remarked: "The observations and classifications of mental disorders has been so exclusively psychological that we have not realized that they

*Controlled, brief fasting, with large doses of the Bulgarian lactobacillus organisms—administered in tablet form or cultures, or by consumption of large amounts of yogurt—has brought significant improvement in mental function for many disturbed children and adults. The procedure must *always* be medically supervised.

illustrate the same pathological principles as other diseases, are produced in the same way, and must be investigated in the same spirit of positive research. Until this is done, I see no hope of improvement in our knowledge of them, and no use in multiplying books about them."

Despite the validity of the warning, the books have multiplied. Whatever their central theses, they almost universally share a philosophy: psychiatric patients have heads, but no bodies. In needed reaction to this obviously unsuccessful approach to psychiatric disorders, a group of determined researchers have been delving into the metabolic disturbances which precede, accompany, initiate, aggravate, or prolong psychiatric illnesses. Oddly enough, the first real breakthrough came over fifty years ago, but was largely ignored, save by a few medical researchers, until I wrote a best-selling book on the subject in the 1960s. I refer to the discovery of low blood sugar (hypoglycemia) by Dr. Seale Harris. Since in this book you will encounter many references to low blood sugar, because it can cause or aggravate most of the symptoms of neurosis and psychosis, it is important that you understand the disorder.

In the 1920s, insulin had been introduced for the treatment of diabetes, and patients and their physicians accepted it as a gallant white knight who would rescue diabetics from the threat of attenuated death. Part of that proved later to be based on an oversimplified view of diabetes as involving only impaired tolerance for sugar, which is but part of the disease; and as *one* disease, which it isn't. Part of it was true, but the rest involved a familiar disappointment, as physicians encountered with insulin what they do with all drugs: side reactions. Medical men were giving uniform doses of this sugar-burning hormone to patients who were not uniform and whose reactions could not be. The result was the discovery of insulin shock—the penalty for an overdose of the hormone, causing the blood sugar to drop too far, too fast, with the patient becoming pale, perspiring, acting incoherent, or falling unconscious. So it was the physicians learned that these patients must be warned to carry identification as diabetics, so that these symptoms, striking without warning, could not cause them to be mistaken for alcoholics.

Seale Harris was wrestling with this problem when, in a moment of medical serendipity, he made a monumental discovery: there were patients who were *not* diabetic, and who, obviously, were *not* using insulin, and yet were indubitably victims of insulin shock. Dr. Harris logically concluded that there are people in whom the pancreas is overactive, and who manage, in response to a rise in blood sugar, to *produce* too much insulin, the effects of which, of course, would be as profound as those of an injected overdose.

One wonders, naturally, why physicians ignored Dr. Harris' discovery for a half-century, surely an aggravated example of the cultural lag for which medicine is notorious. After all, the practitioner is reminded in his daily practice that any gland may be normal, underactive, or overactive—why should the pancreas be thought of only in terms of normalcy or underactivity? For one reason, the warped view obtained because the profession had for too long been preoccupied with diabetes, considered, however mistakenly, to be the toll for the lazy pancreas' underproducing of insulin. Then, too, diabetes is life-threatening, and hypoglycemia rarely is, though its victims may in their protracted agony sometimes wish it were. The symptoms of hypoglycemia also raised the physician's hackles: what validity could there be in the notion that a single disorder could cause anything from claustrophobia to impotence, from anxiety to frigidity—familiar symptoms any M.D. worthy of his stethoscope *knew* were purely emotional. To add to medical unenthusiasm for the concept of hypoglycemia, there was the fact that the treatment was virtually entirely dietetic. Since nutrition was long a subject about which medical men couldn't care less—or in which they couldn't possibly have less training—low blood sugar, however great its contributions to wrecking careers, marriages, and personalities, wasn't a likely candidate for medical screening procedures, the more so because the blood test for diabetes does not identify low blood sugar, diagnosis of which requires a six-hour test, with seven withdrawals of blood—a procedure too demanding and too costly to become a routine segment of the "complete physical examination." To add to the factors encouraging medical suspicion of hypoglycemia, the norms from which the conclusions are drawn are themselves fallacious, derived as they are from a "normal population" which, eating an enormous tonnage of sugar, is anything but normal in its reactions to the test.

To pick up again the story of the pioneering research of Dr. Seale Harris, his next effort was to identify the trigger for this excess production of insulin. Cancer of the pancreas, denominated by Mayo Clinic as the *only* cause of hypoglycemia, is too rare a disease to explain the large number of people obviously suffering from hypoglycemia. The primary trigger proved to be the American accomplishment of eating more than one-hundred pounds of sugar per person, per year. In response to this unhealthy intake of sucrose, the pancreas became oversensitized to it, and responded to small rises in blood sugar with a disproportionate output of insulin. This led to Harris' realization that the *logical* treatment of hypoglycemia—eating sugar to raise blood sugar—would simply lead to more insulin production and less blood sugar, a paradox which also helped to delay medical acceptance of the condition, its causes, and its proper treatment. Logic dictated banning sugar for a diabetic. Would it not insist that a patient with low blood sugar eat more sweets, to raise his blood levels?

While medical men were neglecting or rejecting the concept of hypoglycemia, a few pioneers entered the arena and demonstrated the devastating effects of hypoglycemia on mind and body, and the almost miraculous recoveries which followed prescription of a sugar-free diet, restricted in starch and high in protein and fat. Among these—Portis, Conn, Salzer, Rosenberg, Lee, Tintera, Nittler, and many others—there was a physician who himself suffered from low blood sugar, and vainly visited fourteen specialists and three diagnostic centers, including Mayo Clinic, in an effort to find an explanation for the blackouts which had already involved him in two serious automobile accidents, and for his nervousness, fatigability, irritability, and difficulties in concentration. He emerged from the seventeen diagnostic consultations with a number of verdicts: he was a constitutional inadequate, too frail to stand the stresses of practicing medicine; he was a neurotic; he had (Mayo Clinic said) a brain tumor; his blood vessels were occluded, and circulation to the brain was impaired. He finally arrived at a correct diagnosis, which he made, himself, after reading and acting upon Dr. Seale Harris' paper on hypoglycemia. When a simple change in his diet had wiped out his symptoms, he began to specialize in low blood sugar, treating more than a thousand patients with the disorder. Bitter over his personal experience with medicine's blindness toward hypoglycemia, he wrote a stinging letter to the J.A.M.A., which the journal published in Vol. 152, July 18, 1953. In part, it read:

> If all physicians would read the work of Dr. Seale Harris . . . thousands of persons would not have to go through what I did. During three years of severe illness, I was examined by fourteen specialists and three nationally known clinics before a diagnosis was made by means of a six-hour glucose (sugar) tolerance test, previous diagnoses having been brain tumor, diabetes, and cerebral arteriosclerosis. . . . Since then I have used this hard-earned knowledge in diagnosis and curing the condition in numerous patients.
>
> (Signed) Stephen Gyland, M.D., Tampa, Fla.

For a medical audience at the New York Academy of Medicine, Dr. Gyland delivered a scientific paper on his experience in treatment of hundreds of hypoglycemics, all, like the doctor himself, victims of maldiagnosis, all assured that they were "nervous," "neurotic," or living proofs that disease can in fact be psychosomatic. Neither the local medical society nor the A.M.A. printed that paper; in fact, Dr. Gyland found American medical journals so apathetic to his research, monumental as successful treatment of 1,100 patients with an unrecognized disorder was, that he wasn't able to persuade one of them to publish his report. I secured a copy of it from a Brazilian medical journal, in São Paulo, where it finally appeared—in Portuguese.

It was long after Dr. Gyland left the scene that we arrived at a clearer understanding of the reasons for the hypoglycemic's kaleidoscopic varieties of mental and physical symptoms. Not only is the total brain very sensitive to lack of its prime fuel—sugar—but the emotional brain is even more so. Collateral with the activity of that brain are the centers for control of the autonomic activities of the body—those which, fortunately, continue without our conscious supervision or volition—including the rippling of the intestine, as it moves food along; the beating of the heart; breathing, and many other activities essential to life. Failure of the fuel supply for these centers pushes a panic button.

Don't treat this as a small tempest in a medical teapot. *You* can be told you're neurotic, just as Gyland mistakenly was. *You* can be labeled as a hypochondriac when you actually need a change in diet and in your vitamin supplements, rather than talk-therapy and tranquilizers. *You* can be accused of psychosis and plied with shock therapy and psychotropic drugs when your real need is a reduction in sugar intake and a rise in the supply of nutrients for which your body and brain are pleading. In that context, it is interesting to look at Dr. Gyland's patients, the symptoms of which they complained, the percentage complaining of each symptom, and the mistaken diagnoses they had previously received:

Nervousness	94%
Irritability	89%
Exhaustion	87%
Faintness, dizziness, tremor, cold sweats, weak spells	86%
Depression	77%
Vertigo, dizziness	72%
Drowsiness	72%
Headaches	71%
Digestive disturbances	69%
Forgetfulness	67%
Insomnia (awakening and inability to return to sleep)	62%
Constant worrying, unprovoked anxieties	62%

Mental confusion	57%
Internal trembling	57%
Palpitation of heart, rapid pulse	54%
Muscle pains	53%
Numbness	51%
Indecisiveness	50%
Unsocial, asocial, antisocial behavior	47%
Crying spells	46%
Lack of sex drive (females)	44%
Allergies	43%
Incoordination	43%
Leg cramps	43%
Lack of concentration	42%
Blurred vision	40%
Twitching and jerking of muscles	40%
Itching and crawling sensations on skin	39%
Gasping for breath	37%
Smothering spells	34%
Staggering	34%
Sighing and yawning	30%
Impotence (males)	29%
Unconsciousness	27%
Night terrors, nightmares	27%
Rheumatoid arthritis	24%
Phobias, fears	23%
Neurodermatitis	21%
Suicidal intent	20%*
Nervous breakdown	17%
Convulsions	2%

The patients also commented on changes in personality in the form of unaccustomed lapses in moral conduct, carelessness in dress, and tendencies to drug and alcohol addiction. Despite this evidence (and there is more), the authorities in the fields of drug addiction and alcoholism have not, to this day, investigated the contributions of hypoglycemia in initi-

*A disorder in which 220 patients out of 1,100 are thinking of suicide should be worthy of medical and psychiatric attention, should it not?

ating or prolonging these addictive disorders—and I assure you that hypoglycemia plays a part in some cases of both.

Look back, now, over that list of symptoms.* How could these patients have convinced any physician that they weren't neurotics, any psychiatrist that they weren't ripe candidates for group therapy, psychodrama, tranquilizers, psychic energizers, antidepressants, or a few years on the couch? Many of them *had* been told their symptoms were expressions of neurotic conflicts. Others were (mistakenly) advised that they were victims of various physical diseases, most of which were actually expressions of hypoglycemia, which is almost as great an imitator as syphilis. Only one diagnosis in 600 related to the real disorder—low blood sugar.** Here are some of the erroneous diagnoses:

> Neurosis
> "Slightly nervous"
> Chronic urticaria (hives)
> Neurodermatitis (itching and rash caused by nervousness)
> Ménière's syndrome (loss of hearing, noises in the ears, dizziness associated with these symptoms)
> Cerebral arteriosclerosis (hardening of the arteries of the brain)
> Cephalalgia, hemicrania (pain in the head, or in half the head)
> Psychoneuroticism
> Chronic bronchial asthma***
> Rheumatoid arthritis
> Parkinson's syndrome (palsy)

*A topical note of interest: a star woman athlete, the newspapers recently announced, had finally learned why her playing has slumped. Her physician's diagnosis: hypoglycemia; his prescription: candy bars. It is now almost a half-century since Dr. Seale Harris demonstrated that sugar worsens hypoglycemia.

**Imagine these symptoms added to the dysperceptions and delusions of a schizophrenic, and you will realize why treatment of low blood sugar in psychotics is not an option, but mandatory.

***There is a type of asthma, my research indicates, specifically caused by low blood sugar. When the underlying hypoglycemia is cured, the asthma disappears.

Paroxysmal tachycardia (rapid beating of the heart)
"Imaginary sickness"
Menopause
Alcoholism
Diabetes
Hyperinsulinism (the diagnosis was correct, but the prescription called for candy bars!)

Orthodox medicine persists in declaring functional low blood sugar a very rare disorder, but concedes that it has become a "fad disease"—implying that few of those diagnosed as suffering from it, really do. *Scientific* medical research draws very different conclusions. The medical department of United Airlines tested 177 pilots for low blood sugar, and found 44 cases. One of the pilots remarked that his only symptom was a feeling of confusion when he drove his car in traffic, compelling him to pull over, off the road, and rest for a while. In an examination of 5,000 *healthy* young soldiers, newly inducted into the Army, a physician found, and reported in *Diabetes*, a medical journal, more than 700 cases of low blood sugar. In Part II, where hypoglycemia testing and treatment are described in detail, you will learn that a significant percentage of troubled children and adults, ranging from schizophrenics to the hyperactive and autistic and disturbed, suffer with low blood sugar. So do 60 percent of the patients in average psychiatric practice, as reported in several research papers. As one of the psychiatrists who performed such research remarked, it was frightening to realize how many of the patients he had treated with talk and tranquilizers were suffering from a deficit of fuel in the brain, distorting their perceptions, twisting their thinking and emotions, and interfering with their communication with the practitioner.

The number of cases of hypoglycemia is, if anything, understated. Probably we all have it, most of us as a transient disturbance, but an educated guess would put its incidence in chronic form at one in ten of the general population. That is a conservative estimate, no matter how apoplectic it makes "scientists" who label it as "hogwash" while delivering lectures under the auspices of the manufacturers whose business will most suffer when low blood sugar is diagnosed: makers of junk foods, food additives, cola beverages, and sugar—carefully disguised under the aegis of a foundation representing itself to be a source of unbiased information in nutrition—The Nutrition Foundation.

Why has low blood sugar become so common? To answer that question, we must first realize the complexity of the metabolic controls of the body's slender sugar reserves. (You have less than two teaspoonfuls of sugar in your entire bloodstream, when you haven't eaten for a few hours.) In the brain is a glucose thermostat, turning sugar reserves "on" and "off," exactly like the one that controls the heat or air-conditioning in your home. It gives the signal when the supplies of sugar reaching the brain need adjustment. In response, the body produces HGH, a hormone which raises blood sugar levels, and glucagon, with the same action. The response will, if necessary, elicit production of insulin, to help burn sugar and to recycle reserve supplies, and adrenal hormones, which raise blood sugar and stimulate release (from the liver) of stored fuel. Factors which may interfere with this dynamically balanced mechanism include prolonged stress, caffeine (of which we use more than any other culture), sugar (where our intake ties for first place), poor absorption of sugar, excessively slow or excessively rapid burning of the fuel, or allergies (which afflict more than forty million Americans).

As you examine that list, it becomes obvious that we Americans neglect nothing that might upset our sugar metabolism. We eat 1⅓ teaspoonfuls of sugar, per person, every thirty-five to forty minutes, twenty-four hours per day. We ingest caffeine and related stimulant compounds from coffee, tea, cola drinks, chocolate, cocoa, and stimulant tablets and cold capsules. Our allergies touch off hypoglycemia; our hypoglycemia triggers allergies. The complex dynamics of the sugar-controlling mechanism in the body suggest that it is capable of compensating for temporary metabolic insults, but might seriously be disturbed by conditions Nature could not have anticipated. For example, consumption from soft drinks (daily) of the amount of sugar supplied by twenty-four apples. Nobody eats two dozen apples a day; millions drink that much soda-pop, and more. If one were trying to create hypoglycemia, he would duplicate American nutrition and living habits. To make the possibility of developing the disorder even more certain, add a genetic tendency to diabetes, which is in the background of millions of Americans. Pertinent here is another observation of Seale Harris: the (untreated) hypoglycemia of today becomes the diabetes of tomorrow.

While organized medicine, in chorus with the organized purveyors of sugar-saturated foods and beverages, is decrying hypoglycemia as the "latest fad," consider what happens to people for whom hypoglycemia is a very real disease. A few histories, from the multitude in my files, are typical examples. A young married man, employed as an elevator operator, suffered several blackouts while operating the car. The company physician tested him for epilepsy, couldn't demonstrate it, but nonetheless gave him anti-epilepsy medication. When this failed to stop the attacks, he ordered the young man discharged, as an obviously necessary gesture of protection for the public. Because several blackouts had occurred while the young man was walking on the street, the physician cautioned him to remain at home, lest he be injured in such falls. For a number of years, the young wife worked to support the family, and her husband remained in the apartment, leaving only when his wife was able to accompany him. In the fifth year he began to exhibit signs of delusions of persecution which, under the circumstances, may have been a normal reaction to his strange imprisonment. Since he also lost his libido and became impotent, his wife took him to a clinic, where he encountered a Freudian psychiatrist. The basis for paranoid behavior, in strict Freudian interpretation, is latent or overt homosexuality, which in this case, also served to explain his lack of sexual interest in his wife. Now labeled as an idiopathic epileptic, meaning that his convulsions were of unknown origin, and as a latent homosexual with delusions of persecution, the patient was in real danger of remaining an unsung casualty of the inflexibility of medical and psychiatric dogma. A fortunate accident intervened: the patient had another of his blackouts, and the nearby physician who ministered to him was, by the grace of providence, a specialist in hypoglycemia. (He was, in fact, my co-author in writing my first book on hypoglycemia.) A glucose tolerance test revealed a very severe case of low blood sugar. The diagnosis was confirmed by the results of the treatment, for the hypoglycemia diet, supplemented with ample amounts of brewer's yeast and glycine (an amino acid), produced a dramatic improvement in less than two months, and total recovery in three.

Despite tens of thousands of such responses in the practices of hundreds of physicians and psychiatrists, the hardcore opponents of the basic concepts of hypoglycemia continue to resist the concept. Rarely has the proverbial allergy of medicine to new ideas so devastatingly condemned millions of desperate patients to years of unnecessary suffering. A recent comment from a physician, a specialist in carbohydrate chemistry, is typical of obstructionist tactics calculated to mislead both the public and the profession: "Low blood sugar is meaningless. We can lower the blood sugar with small doses of insulin to one-fourteenth of normal; if we do it slowly, there are no symptoms." There are two key terms in that statement. The adverb *slowly* is meaningless, for it is *fast* drops in blood sugar to which hypoglycemics, by definition, over-react. "Small doses of insulin" is also misleading: it is overproduction of insulin which is the concept behind functional hypoglycemia.

Against such sophistry and chicanery, it is instructive to consider some of the actual statements of hypoglycemics:

A physician, himself a patient, remarked: "Your book [on hypoglycemia] saved my sanity."

A psychologist, herself a patient, said: "It wasn't until I was put on the hypoglycemia diet that I realized that I wouldn't have to learn to live with my symptoms."

An alcoholic said: "I didn't make any vows—I just went

on the diet, and six weeks later realized that I hadn't had a drink in a week—for the first time in forty years—and didn't want one—for the first time in forty years. I am off liquor now for more than three years, after striking out with Antabuse, psychiatric treatments, shock therapy, and tranquilizers.''

The wife of an air force officer wrote: "I was on my way to a sanitarium for shock therapy, to treat the psychosis I developed after our daughter was born, when my husband came across your book. A fine doctor tested me for hypoglycemia, found a very severe case, as he put it; treated it—how successfully, you will know when I tell you these are the first thoughts I've been able coherently to put on paper since the dreadful illness began.''

A captain in army intelligence remarked: "Knowing from your book that sugar makes hypoglycemics worse, I took my wife out of a hospital where, God help us, they were giving her intravenous glucose, which was obviously (to me, not to her doctor) causing her convulsions, and had her tested for low blood sugar. She had a bad case, but she's well, now, for the first time in years. You may be interested to know I came to the hospital from Viet Nam, on compassionate leave—they thought she was dying. I read the book en route from California to Birmingham, and recognized in it more than twenty symptoms my wife had had for years, prior to her hospitalization. She had been told she was a hypochondriac and a severe neurotic. On the diet she is now well.''

The mother of a small boy accused of psychomotor epilepsy, which he didn't have, remarked: "Until I saw one of Jerry's 'fits' touched off by one single bottle of a cola drink, I didn't really believe it could be possible. I'm feeling very guilty now, thinking of all the candy, soft drinks, and cookies I used to feed him. I couldn't believe then that these 'goodies' were giving him attacks of low blood sugar. I've learned my lesson, as has my boy, though it's still difficult to keep him away from sweets, at times.''

From decades of experience as a nutrition educator, I know that the prime problem in persuading the hypoglycemic to change his faulty habits derives from two misconcepts dearly embraced by the public. The first is the belief that the dietary choices shared by 200 million Americans just *can't* be wrong, which is another way of saying that the average *must* be normal. The second, inchoate in the first, is the equally mistaken belief that men are not only created equal, but are biochemically homogeneous. This is to say that we all have the same dietary needs and tolerances, which would automatically excommunicate those who find nothing but troubles in a yearly intake of more than one-hundred pounds of sugar. The fact is that our biochemical differences are greater than our similarities. Jack Sprat does exist. Allergies represent such differences running riot in a clearly visible way, but intolerances to food do exist, and exact a similar—but unrecognized—toll. So it is that there are those who "burn" sugar too fast, and those who burn it too slowly, and those who fall into neither category, but whose cells do not take full advantage of energy sources because the body is not receiving, from an "average" diet, its elevated requirements for energy activators—the vitamins and minerals. For this latter group, a "well balanced" diet is a shibboleth; given that no one in a sedentary civilization can possibly eat an unlimited amount of food, these people can't achieve optimal nutrition from three meals a day, however "well balanced"; their nutrient requirements are too high, and they require supplements of the energy-activators. In two people of the same height and weight, the total energy metabolism is often approximately the same but, as Dr. Roger Williams so ably points out, the details of the burning process may be significantly different. The specific chemical reactions, which are enzyme-dependent and which are involved in the release of energy from food, may take place ten times more rapidly in one person than another. Such differences will, of course, influence their needs for the nutrients vital to the chemistries by which the body manages, at a startlingly low temperature, to "burn" food. These differences show up in studies of the needs for amino acids, the building blocks of proteins, where the range of requirements may vary from person to person by factors up to seven. Calcium requirements may vary by a factor of four; vitamins, by a factor of forty. Tolerance for concentrated sugar, unsurprisingly, may vary, too. You accept that in a diabetic, as you accept the diabetic's need for supplementary insulin. This really commits you to accepting the corollary phenomenon of the hypoglycemic, producing too much insulin, who requires freedom from large doses of sugar, and the addition to his diet of supplements of vitamins and minerals critical to normal release of energy from food. That in turn obligates you to consider the possibility that failure to meet the biochemical needs peculiar to an individual may produce dysfunction, rather than disease: the brain performing at less than its potential, and the personality warped into the less-than-ideal. Williams reminds us that an ounce of yeast, given optimal nutrition, would grow to a million tons in a week. It would fall far short of that increment if grown on citrus juice, a nutrient medium which for yeast represents a compromise. Our nutrition always represents such a compromise. The yeast grown on citrus juice isn't *sick,* and human beings on a suboptimal diet may not be, either; but like the yeast, we adapt to the potential our compromise in nutrition allows us—without realizing that we have compromised, without realizing that our physical and mental functions are thereby falling short of the levels they could achieve.

So it is that there are those who develop or aggravate the symptoms of neurosis or psychosis when they consume, as Americans generally do, an average of $1^1/_3$ teaspoonfuls of sugar every thirty-five minutes, twenty-four hours daily; and others who eat that much sugar with apparent impunity. There are those who are driven into hyperactivity by food additives; others ingest them and go unwounded. As removal of sugar from the diet of the intolerant produces remarkable physical and mental improvement in most hypoglycemics, so does addition of nutrients to a suboptimal diet produce startling responses in others. A researcher comments on a young man whose intellectual function and interests broadened tremendously after he was given 300 mgs. of calcium pantothenate, a B complex vitamin, daily. A *good* diet may supply 10 mgs.

of this factor, which is essential to release of energy from fats. The striking point in this history is the fact that the young man was totally unaware that his intake of this vitamin was the limiting factor in his diet. Such deviants antagonize the establishment in nutrition, which is hopelessly wedded to the concept of a ''standard reference American''—the average consumer who is supposed to thrive on a random selection of highly processed foods laden with additives. There is no room in this philosophy for the deviant who requires better nutrition for optimal mental and physical help.

In Section II, we are devoted to the special needs and the intolerances of the un-average. You will find that the procedures—in dietetic management of hypoglycemia, for instance—seem complex, but they are simpler to follow than describe, and the rewards are out of proportion to the effort. If the extra care rescues you from years of subfunctioning, or from endless psychiatric talk-tranquilizer therapies; if it lets you, perhaps for the first time in your life, achieve your full potential, minus your fears, anxieties, self-doubts, nervousness, irritability, distortions of reality, and weariness, the extra effort will have done for you what it's already accomplished for tens of thousand of *ex*-members of ''The Society of It's All In Your Mind.'' Because sometimes—more frequently than organized medicine, psychiatry, and the food establishment will ever admit—it isn't.

·7·

The Dogs May Bark, but the Caravan Moves On

IN CONTEMPLATING THE proverbial resistance of medicine to new ideas, one is reminded of the prehistoric animal so huge that its tail might successfully be attacked before a neural message could be flashed to the distant brain. It was a fault for which Nature compensated by creating a second brain, at the base of the tail, yielding one of the few creatures genetically equipped for reasoning both *a priori* and *a posteriori*. But for the monster of medicine, no supplementary brain exists, and the creature reacts sluggishly and with marked aversion to changes in its environment.

There is, though, a significant difference between medicine's characteristic resistance to innovation, and the bitter hostility of psychiatry and medicine to the orthomolecular concepts. One senses a grimness in the battle, as though the talk-therapists consider the new approach as a threat to the very survival of the conversation-and-calmative-drugs therapies; and in part, they are right. On no other grounds could one explain the attempt of the orthodoxy in psychiatry to make these innovative and frequently effective treatments *illegal*, which is precisely what they propose. The mechanism they employ was created originally to protect the public from incompetent practitioners. It is the peer review concept, in which a group of physicians police their own profession, reviewing methodology, sitting in judgment on the propriety of the therapeutic modalities and techniques of treatment employed by physicians and psychiatrists. Analogous to a charge of heresy in a churchman is the peer review committee's phrase: "unorthodox" or "unconventional" therapy. The principle is simple and praiseworthy, when properly applied. It is at its best in protecting you against a physician who, without your knowledge, is incorporating narcotics or amphetamines in your vitamin injections. He is exposing you to grave mental and physical harm, not only without your informed consent, but without hope of discernible gain. For such an offense, he may be censured by his peer review organization, or in aggravated offenses, his license may be revoked as an excellent display of the effectiveness of self-policing of the profession for the protection of the public, though it might be well to note that a recent revocation of a license took place only after twenty years of abuse of patients by the offending physician.

That same machinery has now been turned into a fast-moving mechanism for outlawing orthomolecular psychiatry and medicine. The first step was the setting up of a peer review committee standard for "acceptable" psychiatric practice, defined as the use of major and minor tranquilizers and antidepressants, electric convulsive therapy, insulin shock, psychotherapy, psychoanalysis, group therapy, psychodrama, sociodrama, operant conditioning, primal therapy, conditional reflex therapy. (The next time you pass a giant mental institution, you may regard it as a monument to the failure of these techniques to make any appreciable dent in significantly and permanently solving the problems of schizophrenia and other psychoses.) You will note that nowhere in the list does the term "diet" or "nutrition" or "megavitamin therapy" occur, and the omission is deliberate and has far-reaching effects. Let us, for instance, assume that you visit an orthomolecular psychiatrist, suffering from depression and suicidal tendencies. He is aware that 20 percent of the patients with hypoglycemia are suicidally depressed; and you have other symptoms which suggest that low blood sugar may be at least part of your problem. He does not proceed on the basis of this guess, but sends you to a competent laboratory, where you undergo a glucose tolerance test, which confirms the diagnosis. Accordingly, he prescribes the diet and supplements for you, but two weeks later, before your hypoglycemia has had a chance to respond, you commit suicide.

Should your family decide to sue the psychiatrist for malpractice, the peer review standards become the critical issue, for under them, the practitioner used an "unacceptable" or "unorthodox" or "unconventional" treatment. Would it have been acceptable to his peers if the practitioner had dosed you with an antidepressant capable of causing severe damage to the brain and nervous system? Of course. Will the doctor's insurance company defend him if you do commit suicide, and your family sues for malpractice? They will *not,* nor would they be obligated to try. On the other hand, should you benefit by the treatment, and file a claim with your insurance company for your medical bills, they can use the concept of "unorthodox treatment" to evade their responsibility to you; and the peer review committee standard will help them in the evasion. Their computers will be so programmed—in fact, are, right now—that they will regurgitate when faced with a term like "megavitamin therapy" or a diagnosis of "hypoglycemia," or "hair-testing for mineral deficiencies or overload." The interesting, if unbelievable, aspect of this charade, other than its obvious effect in crucifying physicians who opt for helpful, harmless nutritional therapies to replace temporary benefit and risky side effects from powerful drugs, is the fact that your insurance company will dutifully pay all claims for orthodox treatment that *doesn't* help you.

This then is the ploy adopted by the dinosaur to discourage the attacks on its tail. It amounts to outlawing an innovative and frequently rewarding, harmless method of treatment, and to embalming, virtually with the force of the law, the older—and bankrupt—therapies. There are other methods of resistance, sometimes subtle, sometimes unbelievably overt. In giving a paper on orthomolecular treatment of children with learning disabilities, at the Cleveland Child Guidance Center, I first encountered a barrage of hostility from nutritionists wedded to the concept that all anyone needs is a "well-balanced diet." This display of ignorance was followed by a suave display of sophistry by a psychoanalyst, who objected to papers on orthomolecular psychiatry because they are largely "anecdotal" and do not reflect double-blind studies—surely a monumental example of scientific doublethink from a profession wedded to a "science" which has never proved its basic postulates, never could, couldn't possibly perform a double-blind experiment in analysis, and never has.

In a more blatant display of obstructionism, the chief psychiatrist at a Canadian hospital walked into the room of a patient who was being treated (successfully, let's note) for a psychiatric disorder, with orthomolecular methods, and informed the layman that his physician was mistreating him—and followed this by demanding that the officials of the hospital take steps to bar the medical man from the institution. This compelled a team of medical nutritionists and orthomolecular psychiatrists to converge on this distant area of Canada, to protect both the patient and the practitioner from such unwarranted and unethical conduct. The battle was ultimately won by the internist, who would otherwise have been compelled to surrender his psychiatric patients to the ministrations of the talk-shock-drug crew of therapists, which would substitute palliation of symptoms for the chance of a full and lasting recovery from many "mental" disorders.

Another battle was fought in the midwest when Blue Shield didn't want to pay the practitioner for treating his patient's hypoglycemia, and rejected payment for hair analysis as a means of testing for mineral deficiencies. In the courts, both actions were won by Dr. John Baron, a medical nutritionist who has thus set a precedent which will be useful to his innovative colleagues from coast to coast.

Canada was also the scene of yet another pitched battle which began when die-hard physicians, determined to outlaw orthomolecular medicine, requested the government, which closely controls the practice of medicine there, to declare orthomolecular therapies "unconventional" and thereby unacceptable. The government began ponderously to move in that direction, but the patients who had benefited by such treatment reacted violently to the proposal, even to the point of picketing the medical establishment. The tragi-comedy reached its height when the reactionary physicians suddenly realized that they had unlocked a government virus that might infect all their practices, for *every* physician, at one time or another, uses a treatment that could, under a government definition, be considered unorthodox or unconventional. So it came about that the medical men who brought the nose of the camel into the therapeutic tent by inviting the government to intervene in a purely medical matter are now joining with the patients to try to stop the momentum they themselves gave to the forces of reaction.

There are quiet methods of sabotaging innovation in medicine. A typical example is that of a psychiatrist who lets it be known that he practices nutritional therapies, and then denies these modalities to the patients who come in search of them. Still another consists of capitalizing on the cloak of infallibility with which the public invests the physician, and announcing that the vitamin therapies for schizophrenia are both useless and potentially harmful—an announcement which, Dr. Abram Hoffer points out, usually originates with practitioners who have actually never tested the therapy.

To avoid the head-on collisions with orthomolecular men, reactionary physicians attempt to draw the battle lines in a county near a metropolitan area. Thus the peer review standards can be drawn in an area where there are few practitioners; but the code then serves as a precedent, drawn upon when the fight is joined in the larger cities. This maneuver, at the time these lines are written, is being attempted in upstate New York. There are but a few innovative practitioners of psychiatry in that area, and the thinking of the establishment dominates, with the predictable result that the peer review standard outlawing orthomolecular practice may well go effortlessly into effect. The area is, however, the proverbial stone's throw from Westchester and from New York City, and this ploy will give the establishments a useful precedent to cite when the issue arises in the metropolitan areas where a relatively large number of orthomolecular practitioners will leap to the barricades, with a good chance to win their right to treat their patients with any harmless modality that offers possible help.

Cooler heads suggest compromise. One psychiatrist, observing a marked improvement in one of four schizophrenics given vitamin therapy, suggested that his colleagues should remember that physicians are *obligated* to try the new (if harmless) when all the older methods have failed. This still brings up the spectre of vague dangers in nutritional treatment for mental and emotional disorders. The fact that this *is* a red herring redolent of resistance to a new concept can easily be demonstrated. The following are the reports of side reactions to enormous doses of vitamins in the treatment of more than 3,900 patients, as reported by their psychiatrists. Among both adults and children, there were 4 cases of hepatitis in 1,500 patients, which were totally unrelated to the vitamin treatment. In 3 patients of the 3,900 swelling of the feet appeared, and in 2 there was swelling of the face; the symptoms in all disappeared when doses of niacin were discontinued. Two patients receiving this vitamin developed a patchy pigmentation of the arms and armpits, which also disappeared when the dose was stopped. With enormous doses of Vitamin C given to more than 3,000 patients for periods of up to ten years, there were only occasional cases of diarrhea which were dose related, i.e., which disappeared when the dose was lowered. *(No deficiencies in Vitamin B_{12} appeared, though Vitamin C was reported to have destroyed the vitamin in human blood. The observation was made in the test tube, which wasn't reported in the newspaper stories; and blood in the laboratory and that in the patient don't always react alike. In this case, they certainly don't. It might be noted that this report came from a physician who has spent much of his professional life as a witness for a government agency in cases against vitamin manufacturers; and as a professional decrier of vitamin supplements and therapy.)*

All this doesn't say you can't be allergic to a vitamin, or to the traces of solvent used in its manufacture. It doesn't say that the next patient who undergoes vitamin and nutritional therapy for a psychosis may not react with evidences of toxicity. It does say that the treatment is very much safer than the tranquilizer-antidepressant regimes prescribed by those who insist on viewing megavitamins with alarm.

It must be made clear that some physicians and psychiatrists who refuse to try nutritional therapies are simply practicing defensive medicine. They fear malpractice suits, and they don't want to risk the censure of their peers and their peer review committee. One might wish they had more courage, but anyone familiar with the pressure which can be exerted on mavericks by the medical establishment can at least understand their reluctance to invite it.

With regard to the pitched, if silent battle going on behind the psychiatric facade: there is nothing a patient can do about peer review committee standards. There is less he can do about the ways in which insurance company computers react to unsanctioned therapies and innovative methods of medical testing. He has no resources to battle the hospitals, so firmly in the control of the medical establishment, which will not admit a patient diagnosed as being hypoglycemic or in need of megavitamin therapy. But you, the public, do have one effective weapon at your disposal: when behind the open door of the psychiatrist you find a closed mind, no one can stop you from going elsewhere. Nor should you feel that the psycho-nutritionist is, more or less, dumping the problem in your lap, for he is, behind the scenes, very intensely dedicated to the battle against the forces of reaction. As a member of a number of medical societies (and an officer of two which are dedicated to nutrition as a prophylactic and therapeutic component of a holistic approach to troubled patients), I can tell you that every effort is being made to persuade physicians to remember that this is not a war in which all truth is on one side. It is, rather, the classical confrontation in the arena of science, on the basis of which most progress is made.

PART II

·1·

The Why and How of Testing and Treatment for Hypoglycemia

IN ORTHOMOLECULAR MEDICINE and psychiatry, testing and treatment may be complex enough to be confusing to a normal person, and bewildering to those who are emotionally or mentally disturbed. Why so many blood tests? Why does the doctor appear to ignore some of the test results by giving vitamins and other nutrients when the blood levels were within normal range? Why does the physician drip solutions of foods under my tongue? Why did he ask for two table-spoonfuls of hair clippings, and only from the back of my neck? Do I really need three hormone injections a week? Why are my vitamin-mineral supplements different from those the doctor prescribed for my friend, who has exactly the same symptoms I do? Why are our diets different, when we're both suffering from low blood sugar?

As an educator, I've never underestimated the intelligence of the average person, who today is medically sophisticated as never before—and a good thing, too, or he would be even more lost in a medical world he never made. There is nothing about the theories behind orthomolecular testing and treatment that's beyond the layman's comprehension, and I explicitly believe that you'll cooperate more fully and effectively with your physician if you know what's being done, why, and how long it may take for some dividends to accrue from the therapies. To that end, this section of *Psycho-nutrition* is devoted. In it, you will find some repetition of technical points partially covered in the text preceding. I am aware of the repetition. It is deliberate and needed, not only to reemphasize important points and lend clarity by full discussion in the context of this section, but for another good reason. If you, the reader *are* hypoglycemic, allergic, schizophrenic, or in any way suffering from the metabolic imbalances misinterpreted as mental and emotional disorders, you are likely to feel as if you're swathed in cotton batting which makes communication—from you or to you—difficult. As one hypoglycemic, complaining about her physician's impatience, said: "He objects to repeating what he has told us—but if we didn't need the repetition, we wouldn't need his tests and treatments."

Hypoglycemia is a symptom, rather than a disease, but its impact makes normal people behave as if they were severely neurotic or psychotic or hypochondriacal. Obviously, it must make life more miserable for schizophrenics, about half of whom have this condition to complicate their disease and to impede their response to all therapies. Low blood sugar occurs (perhaps frequently) in hyperactive children, and has been reported in autism and in mental retardation. It enters into or it perfectly simulates several types of epilepsy, and it may be a cause or a complication of alcoholism, gastric ulcer, allergy, asthma, migraine headaches, and diabetes.

It must be reemphasized that low blood sugar is *not* caused by lack of sugar in the diet, for civilized man has an oversupply of it (with absolutely no need for one crystal of it in the diet). The average American, nonetheless, swallows $1\frac{1}{3}$ teaspoonfuls of sugar, every thirty-five minutes, twenty-four hours a day. Before you hasten to deny that you consume such a cascade of a bad food, remember that we make or import over one hundred pounds of sugar per person, per year, and somebody, obviously, is eating it. Your tendency is to look only at candy, of which we make nineteen pounds for every living American (and some only half-alive) yearly; and you will point to your chary use of the sugar bowl. You forget that most of our sugar intake is invisible (until it surfaces on your hips). There is sugar added to salt (see the term "dextrose" on the label) and a startling amount in ketchup; there is sugar in canned green peas, in the syrup in which frozen and canned fruits are packed, in salad dressings, in bread—which is at least 8 percent sugar, sometimes 10 percent; in cake, pie, cookies, and breakfast cereals. Some of the new "natural" cereals are over 40 percent sugar—a highly unnatural carbohydrate. A doughnut has up to seven teaspoonfuls of sugar; a portion of apple pie has twelve teaspoonfuls, and served a la mode, has *eighteen* per portion! The antacid you take to relieve the indigestion caused by overdoses of sugar is itself frequently made with it, or coated with it, or both. Your vitamin tablet may have sugar in its formula. Baby foods with too high a sugar content (as in many recipes) may help to create the craving for it. The chart which follows gives you an idea of the tributary sources of the overwhelming tide of sugar which insults the American's digestive tract, glands, nervous system, brain, skin, and eyes.

APPROXIMATE REFINED CARBOHYDRATE CONTENT OF POPULAR FOODS EXPRESSED IN AMOUNTS EQUIVALENT TO TEASPOONFULS OF SUGAR

100 grams = 20 teaspoonfuls = 3½ oz. = 400 calories

Food	Amount	Serving	Sugar Equivalent
Candy			
Hershey Bar	60 gm.	(50¢ size)	7 tsp.
Chocolate cream	13 gm.	(35 to lb.)	2 tsp.
Chocolate fudge	30 gm.	1½ inches sq. (15 to 1 lb.)	4 tsp.
Chewing gum		1 stick	⅓ tsp.
Life saver		1 usual size	⅓ tsp.
Cake			
Chocolate cake	100 gm.	2 layer icing (¹/₁₂ cake)	15 tsp.
Angel cake	45 gm.	1 pc. (¹/₁₂ large cake)	6 tsp.
Sponge cake	50 gm.	¹/₁₀ of average cake	6 tsp.
Cream puff (iced)	80 gm.	1 average custard filled	5 tsp.
Doughnut plain	40 gm.	3 inches in diameter	4 tsp.

Food	Amount	Serving	Sugar Equivalent
Cookies			
Macaroons	25 gm.	1 large or 2 small	3 tsp.
Gingersnaps	6 gm.	1 medium	1 tsp.
Brownies	20 gm.	2 × 2 × ¾ inches	3 tsp.
Custards			
Custard, baked	½ cup		4 tsp.
Gelatin	½ cup		4 tsp.
Junket	⅛ quart		3 tsp.
Ice Cream			
Ice Cream	⅛ quart		5 to 6 tsp.
Water ice	⅛ quart		6 to 8 tsp.
Pie			
Apple Pie	⅙ of med. pie		12 tsp.
Cherry pie	⅙ of med. pie		14 tsp.
Custard, coconut pie	⅙ of med. pie		10 tsp.
Pumpkin pie	⅙ of med. pie		10 tsp.
Sauce			
Chocolate sauce	30 gm.	1 tsp. thick hp.	4½ tsp.
Marshmallow	7.6 gm.	1 aver. (60 to 1 lb.)	1½ tsp.
Spreads			
Jam	20 gm.	1 tablespoon level or 1 heaping tsp.	3 tsp.
Jelly	20 gm.	1 tbsp. level or 1 heaping tsp.	2½ tsp.
Marmalade	20 gm.	1 tbsp. level or 1 heaping tsp.	3 tsp.
Honey	20 gm.	1 tbsp. level or 1 heaping tsp.	3 tsp.
Milk Drinks			
Chocolate (all milk)	1 cup, 5 oz. milk	6 tsp.	
Cocoa (all milk)	1 cup, 5 oz. milk	4 tsp.	

Food	Amount	Serving	Sugar Equivalent
Soft Drinks			
Coca Cola	180 gm.	1 bottle, 6 oz.	4⅓ tsp.
Ginger ale	180 gm.	6 oz. glass	4⅓ tsp.
Cooked Fruits			
Peaches, canned in syrup	10 gm.	2 halves, 1 tbsp. juice	3½ tsp.
Rhubarb, stewed	100 gm.	½ cup sweetened	8 tsp.
Apple sauce (no added sugar)	100 gm.	½ cup scant	2 tsp.
Prunes, stewed, sweetened	100 gm.	4 to 5 med., 2 tbsp. juice	8 tsp.
Dried Fruits			
Apricots, dried	30 gm.	4 to 6 halves	4 tsp.
Prunes, dried	30 gm.	3 to 4 med.	4 tsp.
Dates, dried	30 gm.	3 to 4 stoned	4½ tsp.
Figs, dried	30 gm.	1½ to 2 small	4 tsp.
Raisins	30 gm.	¼ cup	4 tsp.
Fruits and Fruit Juices			
Fruit cocktail	120 gm.	½ cup, scant	5 tsp.
Orange juice	100 gm.	½ cup, scant	2 tsp.
Grapefruit juice, unsweetened	100 gm.	½ cup, scant	2⅓ tsp.
Grape juice, commercial	100 gm.	½ cup, scant	3⅔ tsp.
Pineapple juice, unsweetened	100 gm.	½ cup, scant	2⅗ tsp.

The average intake of 100 pounds of sugar per year is deceptive, like most averages, for there are those who don't consume their share: little babies, calorie watchers, reducers, diabetics, and those who know nutrition or who have consulted a competent dentist or medical nutritionist. This brings the average intake to more than one hundred twenty pounds per year, with sugar thus supplying more than 20 percent of the calories in many diets. In addition to helping to incite vitamin deficiency, hypoglycemia, and diabetes, such a physiologically unhealthy amount of sugar tends, in 70 percent* of its consumers, to increase fasting levels of blood insulin, cholesterol, cortisol, uric acid, and triglycerides. It increases the production of hydrochloric acid and pepsin in the stomach, raises the adhesiveness of blood platelets, and induces the body to part with chromium—a metal needed for proper metabolism of sugar. It is conducive to constipation and to increased stool transit time, which may be implicated in disorders of the digestive tract ranging from hiatus hernia to diverticulosis to bowel cancer. It causes enlargement of the liver and, to a lesser degree, of the adrenal glands, and shrinkage of the pancreas. All this translates into sugar acting as a stress on the organism, pushing the body in the direction of diabetes, coronary heart disease, stroke, gastric ulcer and atherosclerosis.

Common sense alone would tell us that more than one hundred pounds of sugar per year is too much of any one food when it contributes no vitamins, but raises the need for them, to the tune, in the case of Vitamin B_1 (thiamin) of a 90-mg. deficit of that vitamin per year.

All this leads to the ultimate question: if we are so flooded with sugar, why should anyone suffer from *low* blood sugar? This simple question, like so many simple questions, has complicated answers. The mechanisms controlling blood levels of sugar are so intricate that it's more startling when they run properly than when they go awry. Among the known causes of low blood sugar are:

1. The body burns sugar too rapidly, due to overproduction of insulin (the hormone from the pancreas which helps us both to burn and to store and recycle our sugar supply). This condition (hyperinsulinism) is theoretically the opposite of diabetes, though that is an oversimplification. Behind excess production of insulin is a galaxy

*Note that 30 percent of the men tested with high intake of sugar escape most of its adverse reactions. Would you care to play Russian roulette with a sugar cube?

of contributory causes, which may involve sensitization of the pancreas by excess sugar and excess caffeine, or by continued emotional stress, anxiety, and tension; or a genetic tendency toward diabetes, first exhibited as the opposite disorder; or an imbalance of the autonomic nervous systems; or allergy.

2. The symptoms of hypoglycemia may result from excessively slow, rather than rapid, burning of sugar.

3. Slow absorption of sugar from the digestive tract is yet another possibility.

4. Lack of an enzyme, such as sucrase, needed in the utilization of sugar may be responsible.

5. Persistently low levels of blood sugar may derive from a true psychosomatic process. The patient's life-style may involve boredom from a lack of challenge or sense of accomplishment. (This is sometimes misnamed "the tired housewife syndrome" when it appears in women bored with monotonous, tedious, repetitive tasks which offer no sense of achievement.) Here there is a letdown at the emotional brain level, which induces a sit-down strike in the sugar-metabolizing machinery of the body. Since we respond to challenge by recycling our sugar reserves, lack of challenge will have the opposite effect, and the resulting low blood sugar levels will impair the patient's will and physical stamina in doing the unrewarding and yet inescapable tasks against which his emotional brain is rebelling.

6. Allergy to foods, molds, hydrocarbons, and other environmental chemicals may depress the blood sugar, or cause all the symptoms of hypoglycemia even when the blood sugar levels remain within normal range. When allergy is involved, a vicious cycle develops, for low blood sugar triggers or worsens allergies, and allergies induce addiction to the very foods responsible for the troubles. (See Chapters Two and Five).

7. Sensitivity to amino (protein) acids on a genetic basis is a cause of a few cases of hypoglycemia. Babies born with inadequate supplies of enzymes needed for protein metabolism may convulse when fed the offending amino acids, leucine or phenylalanine. Adults

may experience migraine headaches and fatigue based on hypoglycemia caused by such reactions.

8. Smokers sensitive or allergic to nicotine or other products of burned tobacco may develop hypoglycemia and its symptoms.

9. The condition is sometimes caused by lack of glucagon, the hormone which is the antagonist of insulin, produced by the body to raise blood glucose levels.

10. Disturbances of the adrenal glands are involved in hypoglycemia in two ways. It has already been mentioned that these glands may be unable to keep up with the overactivity of the pancreas, i.e., the output of sugar-raising hormones may not keep pace with the excessive output of insulin. This is "relative adrenal failure," relieved when the adrenals are freed of the need to cope with the effects of excessive insulin production. Adrenal failure may be direct, rather than relative, in which case these glands do not recover function when the pancreas quiets down. Specific adrenal therapy is available to augment adrenal production, or to give the glands a relative rest, in which to recover their efficiency.

11. Continuous stress, usually in the form of tension and anxiety, has initiated overactivity both in the adrenals and the pancreas. This also becomes a vicious cycle, for anxiety and tension can cause low blood sugar, and hypoglycemia itself causes feelings of unjustified anxiety.

12. A developmental disturbance, at or near puberty in girls, causes the Morgagni syndrome, resulting in hypoglycemia that doesn't respond to the conventional treatments, but requires special measures. X rays of the skull confirm the diagnosis: the bone is usually too thick, but sometimes abnormally thin.

13. Liver function has been disturbed, usually by improper diet, high in sugar and other overprocessed carbohydrates; or by drugs or alcohol and other toxic substances. This is involved in many types and cases of hypoglycemia, since improper diet is so often the prelude to hypoglycemia. The liver alone is not usually the sole factor, but treatment of low blood sugar cannot be effective if function of this organ is not restored to normal.

14. Glucagon, the hormone produced by the pancreas to

raise blood sugar, may be blocked by excessive production of an inactive type of the hormone, synthe-
sized in the gut.

The symptoms of hypoglycemia are multiple, including
both physical and mental disturbances, for the very good reason that a deficit of sugar strikes directly at the functioning
of the brain and the nervous systems, which all depend on
glucose for fuel. The brain uses 30 percent more than other
tissues; lack of the essential fuel therefore pushes a panic
button. The emotional brain is even more sensitive to lack of
fuel than the thinking brain, with the result that a deficit in
blood glucose causes a bewildering array of "mental" and
"emotional" symptoms, irresistibly suggesting neurosis,
psychosis, or hypochondriasis. Similarly affected is the brain
structure housing the controls for the autonomic activities of
the body, such as the heartbeat, breathing, peristalsis, and
other functions which do not require our conscious control.
So it follows that a deficiency in blood sugar will also cause
physical symptoms, including shortness of breath, acceler-
ated heartbeat or extra systoles, gastric pain, and many more.

Though the preceding statements are not subject to challenge, the medical establishment has rejected the concept of
hypoglycemia as a widespread disorder on the specious
grounds that the term covers a grab-bag of shifting symptoms. You now understand why it does. Those symptoms
have been studied by competent physicians, working with
thousands of hypoglycemic patients. They have demonstrated
that the symptoms can be evoked by feeding sugar, and reversed by a diet low in sugar.

Measuring the amount of sugar in your blood at a given moment is not a test for hypoglycemia, though it might accurately
identify diabetes. Translation: a single blood sugar reading of
300 (twice normal after a meal) is almost certainly proof of
diabetes. But a single blood sugar reading below whatever magic
number the physician has picked as his boundary of normalcy
is meaningless. This is analogous to landing on a strange planet,
sampling the air temperature once, and announcing that the

planet has a "normal temperature." What it was two hours before that moment, or may be two hours after it, is very relevant; so with blood sugar. Hypoglycemia is the result of a disturbance in the *dynamics* of the body's management of sugar, and it is thereby established by watching sugar in motion, not standing still. As one can't establish poor utilization of gasoline by a car when its motor isn't running, or guess at it merely by checking the gas gauge, so one can't identify hypoglycemia by a single test of the blood sugar level at a given moment. (Forgive the belaboring of the point, but I have seen too many misinterpretations of sugar-tolerance tests.) To demonstrate the presence of hypoglycemia, the physician must watch what happens after a large oral dose of sugar, observing not only the levels reached in the blood, but the speed with which changes take place and, which is equally important and often neglected, how the patient reacts when the blood sugar sinks *quickly.* This is a most important point: if the patient is a well person, and you bring blood sugar down very slowly, you can drop it almost to the vanishing point, with no symptoms developing. If the person is a true hypoglycemic, a fast change in blood sugar levels will make him ill, and it matters not where the starting point or where the finishing point of the blood glucose changes. If a diabetic takes an overdose of insulin, to reduce his abnormally elevated blood sugar, and reduces the blood level too fast, he is likely to go into shock, though his blood sugar at no time drops below the normal range. Thus a *fast* drop from a blood glucose of 500 (too high) to one of 150 (normal after a meal) may put a diabetic into a coma; and a *fast* drop in the blood sugar of a hypoglycemic, say from 150, normal after a meal, to 75, normal fasting level, will cause just as much trouble. I have watched severe hypoglycemic reactions, including obvious insulin shock and convulsions, in a sufferer who during the test never showed a blood glucose below 77—well within the range physicians are taught to count as normal; and so has any laboratory technician who has observed a number of glucose tolerance tests. Elsewhere, I have told the story of a patient whose blood glucose, during the test, tended toward prediabetes (177) but dropped into the low 50's in several hours. The test was called normal although the patient, during its course, convulsed, stuttered, and lost all color vision. As an experienced baby nurse has been heard urging parents to "put down the Spock, and pick up the baby when he cries," so does the medical nutritionist put down the glucose-tolerance test, and watch the patient's reactions. This explains my emphasis on a rule which must be observed: a competent attendant, if not the busy physician himself, should always be in the room where the glucose test is given, for severe reactions can and do appear, and some of them may occur after hours of testing have yielded nothing significant, either in the glucose levels or in the patient's prior responses to them. For the same reason, it is very important that you report to the physician *every* subjective reaction you experience during the test. Events invisible to the physician may have profound significance. A headache during the test has as much meaning as a coma—particularly when headaches have been one of your constant problems. A feeling of confusion, out of the blue, is meaningful. So is an unprovoked attack of anxiety, with a sensation of "something terrible about to happen." Such symptoms should be noted, and the observations transmitted to the doctor.

The most widely used method of testing for hypoglycemia involves a study of the blood glucose levels at six intervals after a dose of sugar, administered when the stomach is empty, has been swallowed, with a preceding test of the fasting level of glucose. The doctor will observe whether, in response to the dose of sugar, the blood level rises as it should. Ideally, it should increase by about 50 percent over the fasting level, and no more than 100 percent. When 50 percent over the fasting level is achieved, and the resulting figure is below a functioning level for the brain and nervous systems (indicating, of course, that the starting point itself was too low), the physician will take this into consideration in making his diagnosis. No symptoms should be caused by the test. Drops of more than 25 mgs. in any one-hour period should not evoke any reactions in the patient, and the terminal figure in the sixth hour of the test should roughly have fallen to the initial (fasting) level. Surprisingly, if it falls below that, even by what would seem an insignificant amount, it is regarded as at least "latent hypoglycemia," and is treated—which, in patients with symptoms of low blood sugar, may yield astonishing dividends in improved well-being.

What of the patient whose blood glucose does drop more than 25 mgs. in a one-hour period, or whose terminal figure is significantly below his fasting level, but who is symptom-free? The medical voices which belittle hypoglycemia (in the most ignoble tradition of medicine, which has belittled *every* new discovery in the field) describe such patients as suffering from "chemical hypoglycemia," which means they are symptom-free and hence not deserving of treatment or continued scrutiny. One need not be a physician to remember that detection programs for diabetes are aimed specifically at those who are *symptom-free*, but do have elevated blood glucose, denoting diabetes. Otherwise, why are detection programs needed? This is chemical (as distinguished from clinical) diabetes, and you can bet your sweet lollipop that these patients aren't told they should go home and forget the whole thing. Which makes it bitterly inexcusable that those with chemical hypoglycemia should be told to ignore the condition—particularly when untreated low blood sugar, with or without symptoms, may be a prelude to diabetes. Not at all incidentally, it's perfectly possible to have both disorders simultaneously, diabetes and hypoglycemia, with the blood sugar alternating between excessively high and excessively low levels. Here the competent physician will treat the conditions as one entity, rather than two opposed diseases: as disturbed carbohydrate metabolism, prescribing the regime he would use for hypoglycemia alone.

The preceding remarks indicate that interpretation of the results of the sugar-tolerance test has also become, gratuitously, a storm center. Another focus of debate is the length of the test. Many patients display a normal reaction in the first two or three hours, but develop symptoms later. Though they are commonly used, one-hour or two-hour tests, though they may confirm the presence of diabetes, frequently show no evidence of low blood sugar, which may not appear until the fifth or sixth hour of the test. (I once saw a patient convulse in the sixth hour; had the doctor sent her home at the fifth hour of the test, he would have assured her that she did not have hypoglycemia.) A six-hour test is likely to be accurate.*

Those who regard the average American on his average diet as well-fed and healthy are automatically led into another trap when interpreting the glucose-tolerance test. They point out that routine glucose-tolerance tests in average Americans will reveal thousands of variations from the theoretical norm; such reactions, they insist, are normal—because they are *average*.

The question which is begged here is obvious: what's normal? Can you accept as such the reactions of millions of Americans who torture their bodies with more than 100 pounds of sugar per year—an intake impossible to achieve from natural sources in any conceivable diet that might support good health? This is analogous to declaring pyorrhea and periodontal disease as normal, on the grounds that they're certainly average—over 80 percent of all Americans over the age of thirty-five have disease of the gums and the supporting structures of the teeth. Would this mean that the American without loose teeth, infected gums, and decalcified jawbones is unhealthy? To get away from this kind of "logic" we might note that the National Institutes of Health has estimated that a large majority of Americans show abnormal glucose tolerance.

The fact that a large dose of sugar touches off hypoglycemia and its panoply of symptoms doesn't necessarily guarantee that sugar itself is the mischief-maker, though it probably is, in the majority of cases. Sometimes, though, the patient may be reacting allergically to the *source* of the sugar, with the allergy causing hypoglycemia and its symptoms. The glucose given in a tolerance test is derived from acid treatment of corn, and a pound of glucose could contain as much as one-thirtieth of an ounce of corn protein. If you are exquisitely sensitive to corn,

---

*The accuracy of the six-hour test may be improved if the patient exercises or hyperventilates after the fourth-hour sample of blood has been drawn. This stress may bring a very sharp drop in blood glucose and elicit symptoms of hypoglycemia which otherwise may not have appeared. In apparently normal individuals, the stress test has sometimes caused outright symptoms of schizophrenia to appear.

as some people are, a dose of glucose may light the fuse for an explosive allergic reaction to corn itself. If you are sensitive to beets, from which commercial sugar is often extracted, allergy to beets rather than intolerance to sugar may be the problem. So it is that the orthomolecular practitioner, dedicated to the uses of the right molecules, may have to search for the wrong ones by testing for allergies of the type which have impacts on the brain and nervous systems, for such neuroallergies are potent sources or intensifiers of the symptoms of neurosis and psychosis. Amazingly, such neuroallergic reactions may trigger learned behavior, which is to say that a man who hates his mother-in-law may experience rage against her after he has eaten something to which he is allergic.

The testing of neuroallergies doesn't rest on the familiar scratch and patch tests, reactions to which tend to be localized. They are based more upon your subjective reactions when a solution of the food is dropped under your tongue, where the rich vascular (blood vessel) network will carry it swiftly into the body. If you react badly to such a test, you may be astonished when you find yourself suddenly sleepy, confused, angry, irritable, depersonalized, disorientated, or suffer body-wide aches, pains and spasms which you were previously assured, perhaps, were purely psychosomatic. You will also be startled when the physician negates the symptoms by having you swallow a very dilute dose of the solution which initially caused the reaction. For reasons not well understood, this blocks the symptoms of the allergy. (I have previously pointed out that this antidotal effect of a second dose is the beginning of addiction to the very foods to which you are allergic. Dose #1 stimulates the nervous system, which is at least subconsciously pleasant. When the price for the stimulation is due—the irritability, fatigability, or whatever your allergic reaction—you are addictively driven into repeating ingestion of the food; and the second dose acts as an antidote for the first. Being too large a dose, however, it, too, would exact a price—if you didn't indulge in dose #3; and so on, ad infinitum.) This explains why the favorite foods of allergic individuals are the most suspect of causing trouble. And the trouble may seem so remote from an allergic reaction that psychiatrists may (and usually do) misdiagnose it as a neurotic or psychotic symptom. To credit this fully, you must hear, as I did, a neuroallergist describe a quiet, placid schizophrenic whose behavior seems normal until (unknown to him) he is given a small dose, in another and well-tolerated food, of something to which he is neuroallergic. Within twenty minutes, he is seized by megalomania, announcing that he is the reincarnation of Jesus, but after an antidotal dose of Vitamin C and Vitamin B_6, he again is quiet and his behavior normal. Similar reactions have been traced to sugar derived from beets—not because of the sugar, but because of a beet allergy; and to beer, not because of the beer itself, but the grains from which it was brewed.* You may with justice decide that tests for allergy are an important part of the investigation of the wrong molecules in your system.

Dr. Herman Goodman and I conducted years of research in an effort to shorten the six-hour glucose tolerance test, and still to preserve its accuracy. We were primarily interested in a more convenient screening device for large groups of patients. We finally arrived at a one-hour test which, with some limitations, does a good screening examination. This involves testing the fasting level of blood glucose before breakfast. The patient then eats his accustomed meal and, an hour later, the test is repeated. If the level has not risen by 50 percent and you have definite symptoms of hypoglycemia, the need for the longer test is obviated. If the result is negative and yet you do have symptoms of low blood sugar, the physician may then elect to revert to the longer method.

Still another technique is the device of following you, in terms of blood glucose, through your normal meals and normal day. You are tested before and after breakfast, in midmorning, and before and after lunch. This lets us observe your blood glucose levels as they react to your accustomed

---

*Reactions to milk, though frequent, do not always reflect allergy. They are sometimes caused by deficiency of an enzyme, lactase, needed to break down lactose, which is milk sugar. There are tests for such enzyme deficiency.

meals and pattern of living, with its stresses. Since this test continues into early afternoon, it is pertinent to note that some hypoglycemias which remain hidden in the morning become clearly evident in the latter part of the day. Such a response indicates that the biological clocks of the body are in part determining your reactions to the sugar in your meals. Each of us marches to the beat of a different drum. . . .

The rigors of the long test, and the sometimes severe reactions to it, have induced some physicians to seek a less trying method. The simplest, though regarded as less "scientific," is therapeutic diagnosis. This is a complex term for the simple procedure of placing the patient on the hypoglycemia diet for about six weeks and watching the responses, which has its virtues, particularly for children, since it spares them six or seven withdrawals of blood. The test is interpreted retrospectively: if the patient improved after following the diet, he had hypoglycemia; if he didn't respond, no harm was done, since the diet represents good nutrition for anyone.* The disadvantage of the method is the fact that it doesn't entirely close the door on the possibility of hypoglycemia, even if there is no response to the diet (or even an intensification of symptoms). Possibly, the patient is allergic to some of the permitted foods and would improve if they were eliminated, for they can touch off a drop in the blood sugar and the consequent symptoms, or be responsible for the reactions characteristic of hypoglycemia, even if the blood sugar levels do not change. It might be that the dietary treatment would fail, or at least give only partial relief because this patient needed more carbohydrate and less fat than the usual low blood sugar diet provides. No two people are alike in dietary needs and tolerances, and not everyone is gaited for a limi-

---

*Some physicians regard "therapeutic diagnosis" as unscientific, but it is not an unprecedented use of the technique. If the medical man is not sure whether gout is part of your troubles with arthritis, he may give you colchicine. Since this medication is of benefit only in gout, he knows, if it helps you, that gout is at least one of your problems. This, too, is therapeutic diagnosis.

tation to 60 grams of starch daily, though it is a reasonable starting point for testing.

Conversely, an improvement may sometimes be difficult to interpret. It can, of course, come from normalization of the body's management of sugar metabolism; and usually it does. But it could also derive from better nutrition, or from the fact that the diet minimizes the intake of food additives, of which we now consume per person, per year, more than five pounds, in the form of some 2,700 chemicals—some of them *known* to alter behavior in animals and to contribute to hyperactivity in children. They obviously perform no service, at the very least, for nervous, irritable, emotionally tortured hypoglycemics or sufferers with neuroallergy.

The hypoglycemia diets prescribed by physicians are as low as possible in sugar, which isn't any easy goal when it is an ingredient in so many processed foods, and a natural constituent of many others. Contrary to popular belief, excessive intake of ''natural'' sugar is as harmful to a hypoglycemic as the sucrose in the sugar bowl. The ''fruit sugar'' of fruits, and the content of it in honey are specifically damaging to hypoglycemics; in fact, it is the fruit sugar which is half the molecule of ordinary sugar that makes the latter undesirable. So *all* sugars from *all* sources must be limited. Caffeine is forbidden, tabooing the cola drinks, coffee, tea, chocolate, and cocoa, for this drug stimulates the liver into releasing stored sugar; and when that glycogen reaches the blood as glucose, the overactive pancreas will react to it, which is to say that the organ can't distinguish between your eating a candy bar, or your raising your blood sugar by drawing on your reserves. Alcoholic beverages react adversely on hypoglycemics, who can become very intoxicated or very sleepy with a small intake. Here we must be cautious in interpreting the reaction, for malnutrition, hypoglycemia itself, or allergy to the source of the drink may be responsible for hyper-reactivity to alcohol. If it takes very little liquor to intoxicate the drinker, we grow suspicious of low blood sugar or allergy, one possibly causing or aggravating the other. It is not astonishing, therefore, that some alcoholics lose their desire for hard liquor when hypoglycemia is arrested, exactly as hypoglycemics who are under control tend to lose their craving for sweets.* It follows that arresting low blood sugar will sometimes allow a confirmed alcoholic to take one or two drinks, and stop—which is tantamount to a cure of a condition which has always been treated as a psychiatric disorder.

Since the prime objective of the hypoglycemic diet is to minimize swift ascents and consequent sudden drops in blood glucose, it is necessary to divide the menus into six small, rather than three large, meals daily. These frequent feedings are at least as important as the composition of the menus, for low blood sugar simply can't be controlled if intervals between meals are too long. The diet not only helps to regulate blood glucose, but is helpful in weight control and weight loss, for the body is less efficient in utilizing small meals. Blood cholesterol and triglycerides, as well as blood uric acid, are easier to regulate when the meals are low in sugar and served in more frequent, smaller units.

With these menus, the orthomolecular practitioner will usually prescribe multiple vitamins, trace minerals, and Vitamin B complex supplements from such sources as liver or yeast, if allergies to these foods, which are frequently allergenic because of the large number of factors they contain, do not forbid. Sometimes the physician will advise consumption of liver and yeast only once every four days, to minimize such allergic reactions. The game is worth the candle, for these concentrates not only compensate for the good foods displaced from your former menus by your excessive intake of sugar and other highly processed foods, but they also help in restoring liver function.

A special problem of hypoglycemics is a peculiar type of insomnia. The patient has little difficulty in falling asleep, but tends to awaken in the small hours of the night and has

---

*You now know that there can be an addiction to foods and beverages to which you are allergic. Consider the possibility that the alcoholic is allergic to—and thereby addicted to—either the alcohol itself, or the traces in it of the grains or other foods from which it was made. His craving for the next drink may be clear exhibition of the addictiveness allergics exhibit to the very foods or beverages to which they are adversely reacting.

no success in returning to sleep. The physician, to cope with the drop in the blood sugar, long after the last meal or snack, which triggers the awakening, may suggest that you keep a high-protein beverage at your bedside, and train yourself to awaken and consume it around midnight or 1:00 A.M. You will learn ultimately to do this by reflex, returning to sleep immediately and often sleeping right through the night.

The doctor may also tell you to take a tablespoonful or two of chemically pure glycerin, in water, one to three times daily between meals. In most people, this is converted directly into stored sugar (glycogen) and thereby adds to the reserve on which the body can draw when it needs it. Because of this phenomenon, glycerin usually doesn't stimulate the pancreas, since there is no appreciable rise in circulating blood sugar. The drug may prove too laxative, a reaction which is controlled by lowering the dose. On the other hand, many hypoglycemics are grateful for the laxative effect, which derives harmlessly from the action of glycerin in bringing water into the lower colon.

The ''flat curve'' type of hypoglycemia, which has been previously described as sometimes originating with a flat lifestyle that offers no challenge, will sometimes revert to a more normal curve if the glycerin therapy is used. Another helpful hint some physicians will give in this type of hypoglycemia is an hour of rest after breakfast, even if this requires rising earlier. It seems to help in aiding the body to profit by the glucose in the meal, and particularly in increasing the storage of glycogen, which the glycerin treatment abets.

In all types of hypoglycemia, the doctor may employ medication, usually of the belladonna type, to slow the absorption of sugar from the digestive tract, so that sharp rises in blood glucose do not challenge the overactive pancreas. He may recommend frequent eating of avocado for its content of mannoheptulose, an oddity among sugars, which not only does not stimulate the pancreas, but may actually depress insulin production.

After prescribing the diet, many physicians will simply watch and wait, appraising the effects, for a large majority of hypoglycemics will respond dramatically to the diet and supplements alone. In those who do not respond, or who do so only partially and then strike a plateau, the doctor may institute additional treatment. This may include psychotherapy for those with the flat glucose curve, for no diet or medication will support indefinitely a normal sugar response in those whose difficulty is a feeling of non-accomplishment and lack of challenge. For others, the physician may use injections of adrenal cortex extract. This is based on the need to fortify the action of the adrenals, which have been attempting to raise the blood sugar in the face of persistent efforts by the pancreas to keep it low. In the majority of patients, the adrenals have lost the battle, but are still functionally normal, and will take up their normal duties efficiently as soon as the pancreas stops challenging them with overproduction of insulin. In others—perhaps 10 percent of the hypoglycemics—the adrenals have taken so much stress that they are no longer capable of full recovery even when the pancreatic challenge is removed, and in these cases the injections of adrenal cortex serve to give these glands the rest they need for full recovery from the ordeal.*

Though a hair test in a hypoglycemic may show a high content of sodium, and the blood level may be within normal range, the patient may profit by increased intake of salt and other sodium sources. The physician knows that what is in the hair is being excreted; it is lost to the body, and therefore not necessarily indictive of an oversupply; the sodium (salt) in the blood and hair may not be a reflection of what's reaching the cells, which happens frequently to be true of sodium in a hypoglycemic.

In alcoholism and in the malnourished, the blood sugar may

---

*This type of treatment has been criticized by the medical establishment on the specious grounds that adrenal cortex injections supply only a trace of cortisone. The objection is more than frivolous; it is, if seriously proposed, ignorant, for there are about fifty hormones in the adrenal cortex, the production of which sharply increases when the body is under stress. Since Nature doesn't play games without prizes, it is obvious that injections of adrenal cortex, with its many stress-responsive hormones, are more rational than cortisone therapy alone, for those whose glands have been subjected to the unremitting stresses of hypoglycemia and the insults, emotional and dietetic, which brought it on. Gauging the value of adrenal cortex injections by their cortisone content is analogous to appraising a multiple vitamin concentrate on the basis of its content of just one vitamin.

remain persistently low, despite a corrected diet, frequent feedings, and supplements aiding in correction of liver function. Here the physician may have to turn to intravenous feeding of protein, which, if the liver isn't irreparably damaged is usually successful in raising blood glucose to a functional range.

If you're overweight and hypoglycemic, the doctor will reemphasize the importance of taking 20 percent of your total fat intake in the form of vegetable (polyunsaturated) fats. For complex reasons, such fat not only accelerates the weight loss when it is part of a low carbohydrate diet, but also aids in keeping blood cholesterol down. The same diet, please note, with the same amount of unsaturated fat, will *not* cause weight loss in those who don't need it. The direction of good nutrition is toward the normal.

If you're hypoglycemic and allergic, or schizophrenic, allergic, and hypoglycemic, which are not unusual combinations of troubles, the physician will test you for allergies, and exclude from your internal and external environments as many as possible of the troublemakers. To minimize reactions to those sensitizing foods you can't totally avoid, he may arrange your diet on a four-day, five-day, or six-day rotation basis, so that you have freedom from or long intervals between consumption of disturbing foods. Such rotation not only quiets allergies, but tends to minimize the development of new ones. Large doses of Vitamin C and Vitamin B_6—a gram of each—may be prescribed to offset allergic reactions which sneak by these safeguards. If your allergies are so multiple and intractable that a properly balanced ordinary or hypoglycemia diet becomes almost impossible to attain, your doctor may place you on a fast, during which you consume only pure water. Foods are then restored one at a time, and a rotation schedule is employed. This procedure detoxifies you, in terms of your body's exposure to allergenic foods, and identifies mischief-makers with a high degree of accuracy.

Finally, if the diet suited to your hypoglycemia doesn't quiet your symptoms as expected, and elimination of allergens lends no further help, your physician may increase your intake of complex starches, and lower your gross intake of fats. Some people thrive on 80 grams of carbohydrates a day, but remain tired and nervous below that figure. Some need 100 grams. Some profit by higher intake of fat; some by lower. A typical 60-gram diet follows:

BEFORE BREAKFAST: Use your blender or beater to mix 1 tsp. each of dry skim milk powder, mildly sweetened protein powder, primary food brewer's yeast powder, 2 tsp. of glycerin in water, unsweetened fruit juice, or fluid skim milk. Add any flavoring (vanilla, for example) that pleases your palate. Never miss this supplement; it is a critical part of the dietetic procedure. If for any reason you must skip a meal or a snack as recommended by the diet, take a couple of ounces of this drink. It is only for emergencies; skipping scheduled food is not recommended.

BREAKFAST

Fruit or juice (4 oz.)
1 egg
1 oz. meat or meat
   substitute, such as
   cheese or fish
½ slice whole-wheat
   bread with one
   teaspoon soft
   margarine

1 cup weak tea,
   sweetened
   artificially if desired

MORNING SNACK

1 cup skim milk,
   flavored, if desired,
   with vanilla or other
   sugar-free natural
   flavor

1 oz. meat or meat
   substitute (see
   recipes)

LUNCH

3 oz. meat (cooked
   weight) or meat
   substitute
1 serving vegetables
1 slice bread with 1 tsp.
   margarine
   Green salad with
   cottonseed oil or
   mayonnaise (1 tsp.)

Dessert from approved
   selection (see
   following recipes)
Weak tea or artificially
   sweetened soft drink

Note: A second vegetable may be selected from the list proposed
   as bread substitutes.*

AFTERNOON SNACK

2 oz. meat or meat
   substitute (see snack
   recipes)
½ cup skim milk,
   flavored if desired

½ slice bread with small
   amount margarine

DINNER

3 oz. meat or substitute
   Vegetable
   Green salad,
   cottonseed oil or
   mayonnaise dressing

1 serving approved fruit
   Approved dessert
   Tea (weak) or other
   approved beverage

EVENING SNACK

½ cup skim milk,
   flavored if desired

1 oz. meat or meat
   substitute (see
   recipes)

*Bread substitutions: a half-slice of bread may once daily be replaced by
a half cup of any of the following vegetables: beets, pumpkin, carrots,
onions, peas, rutabaga, turnips, or winter squash.

SUGGESTIONS FOR BETWEEN-MEAL SNACKS

These snacks are all high in protein, though it is possible, of course, to use up some of the allotted bread intake at these little meals. To keep low the amount of carbohydrates from bread, one can use brown-rice cakes, which are available in health-food stores. These weigh half as much as slices of bread, and, when prewarmed, are quite palatable, satiate the craving for carbohydrates (which will lessen as the low-sugar diet is followed) at the snack time, and provide a vehicle for the protein foods.

Note that snack portions are 1 ounce.

COTTAGE CHEESE: a frequent choice of those on the hypoglycemia diet, can be made more palatable by adding chopped dill, chopped chives, chopped onion or scallion, shredded spinach, poppy seeds, caraway seeds, or horseradish.

HAM HORN: Press pot cheese through strainer. Add enough yogurt to make a soft paste and a little chopped dill pickle. Roll this in a paper-thin piece of ham, securing it with a toothpick to make a small horn.

TONGUE-CHEESE HORN: Fill paper-thin tongue slice, rolled into horn shape, with Neufchâtel cheese.

DOUGHLESS PIZZA:

½ lb. lean beef
1 pinch pepper
2 fresh tomatoes
1 medium onion
¼ small can tomato
    paste

⅛ tsp. each of sweet
    basil, oregano, pa-
    prika

Pepper meat and knead. Line small Pyrex dish with meat as substitute for pizza shell. Chop tomatoes with onion and mix with tomato paste and flavoring. Fill meat shell with mixture. Add a touch of oregano on top and bake to preferred doneness at 350°.

TUNA IN CUCUMBER: Hollow out ½ cucumber, stuff with 1 oz. tuna fish mixed with 1 tsp. mayonnaise.

CHEESE FOR SNACKS: These should not be restricted in variety. Use Brie, American, cheddar, pot, farmer, cottage, and be wary only of cheese *spreads,* for these may be diluted with cornstarch or other carbohydrates. Gouda, Swiss, and processed cheese (Velveeta and others of this type) are all good choices. The cheese, for variety, may be combined with another protein: ham as a blanket for a piece of Gouda is delightful, and good nutrition, too.

CELERY STICK AND POT CHEESE (1 oz.): Press cheese through strainer. Moisten it with a small amount of yogurt, buttermilk, or skim milk. Flavor it with chopped green pepper, watercress, parsley, or pimiento, chopped fine. Fill celery stick with mixture.

SNACK BEVERAGE: Take ½ cup plain yogurt (fruit varieties contain an unbelievable amount of sugar) and fizz it in tall glass with carbonated water (club soda) or carbonated mineral water.

STUFFED EGG SNACK: Mash hard-cooked yolks of 3 eggs until fine and crumbly. Add 1 oz. melted margarine, ⅛ tsp. salt, dash pepper; ⅛ tsp. prepared mustard, ½ tsp. minced onion, ⅙ cup flaked tuna, cut-up shrimp, or crabmeat. Mix until smooth, and fill hollows in egg whites, garnishing with slices of olive, pimiento, or parsley. Yields 6 stuffed-egg halves. Reducers should eat only one.

SNACK DESSERT AND BEVERAGE: Pour a little low-calorie ginger ale over 2 tbs. of nonfat milk powder. Use rest of soda as beverage.

CHEESE-APPLE SNACK: Combine a wedge of Gruyère cheese with ½ small apple.

CHICKEN SNACK: Spread 1 oz. of commercial chicken-spread on thin whole-wheat cracker.

KOSHER SNACK: Broiled beef fry—1 oz. of beef (smoked beef plate, used instead of bacon in orthodox Jewish diet). Beverage: V-8 vegetable juice cocktail or equivalent.

YOGURT SNACK: Plain yogurt (4 oz.), with vanilla or almond extract to taste.

COLESLAW SNACK: 1 oz. sliced meat, such as roast beef or tongue, rolled and filled with coleslaw.

SHRIMP SNACK: Commercial frozen shrimp cocktail (1 oz. portion for reducers) is a convenient snack food, very rich in protein. So are canned smoked oysters.

MUSHROOM SNACK: Stuffed mushrooms (2 oz.) filled (topped) with paste made from pot cheese, curry powder, and salt or salt substitute.

PEAR SNACK: Partially scoop out small pear and fill with 1 oz. soft Camembert cheese.

HAMBURGER: 1 oz. ground chuck, with a touch of garlic, 1 tsp. tomato juice, and a dash of tarragon. Broil.

DESSERT SUGGESTIONS

ARTIFICIALLY SWEETENED CUSTARD

3 eggs, slightly beaten
2 cups liquefied nonfat milk
Sweetener equivalent two teaspoonfuls sugar

1 teaspoonful vanilla
Nutmeg to taste

Combine milk and sweetener. Scald in top of double boiler. Add to eggs. Stir in vanilla. Pour into custard cups and sprinkle with nutmeg. Place in pan of hot water reaching within ½-inch of edges of cups, and bake in 300-degree oven until knifeblade in center emerges clean. Usually requires one hour—less if hot water pan is not used. Chill. Serves four.

BLACK CHERRY COUPE

1 envelope unflavored whole gelatin
1½ cups sugar-free carbonated black cherry soda

½ cup cold water
1 cup black cherries, fresh or (sugar-free) canned

Pour water in top of double boiler, sprinkle in gelatin, and stir over hot water until it dissolves. Remove from range, add soda pop, blend. Pour gelatin mixture over fruit in four sherbet glasses. Chill until firm. Serve with small topping of sugar-free whipped cream, which may be "sweetened" with a little vanilla.

QUICK AND REFRESHING FIZZES

Pour sugar-free ginger ale over a few teaspoonfuls of nonfat milk powder, or mix the ginger ale with an equal amount of liquid skimmed milk. When dry powder nonfat milk is used, the dessert is eaten with a spoon. Another quick and refreshing dessert is made with a few large strawberries, blended with a half-cup of skimmed milk. Please remember, though, that milk contains about as much sugar (lactose) as it does protein, and deduct such a dessert from the skim milk allowance in the menus.

WHOLE GELATIN DESSERTS

Commercial preflavored gelatin desserts are 85% sugar with artificial flavor, color, and, frequently, preservatives. Prepare your own gelatin desserts from whole (100%) gelatin, adding permissible fruits, vanilla, or other flavorings to taste. Since gelatin is a rich source of glycine—an amino acid of special importance to some hypoglycemics—such desserts are nutritionally useful to them.

ZABAGLIONE

2 egg yolks
½ cup orange juice
20 grains of saccharin
    crystals

Dash of cinnamon and
    nutmeg

In double boiler, beat egg yolks until thick and lemon-colored. Place over heat, gradually adding orange juice with constant beating until dessert reaches consistency of heavy cream. Add cinnamon, beat briefly, top with ground nutmeg before serving, either hot or cold.

COFFEE WHIP

Sweetener equivalent 2
    teaspoonfuls sugar
1 cup very cold water
2 teaspoonfuls instant
    coffee powder.
    Note: *must* be decaf-
    feinated.

1 egg white
½ cup nonfat dry milk
    powder

At slow speed, electrically beat ice water and nonfat milk until blended. Add sweetener (in liquid form) and instant coffee (powder form). Now mix at high speed until fluffy and light. Add egg white, beat one minute more. Place mixture in six half-cup molds, and freeze for four hours, until firm. Loosen cream with knife edge and tap out of mold. Serves six. Remember that the nonfat milk per portion of this dessert is equal to about ¾ of a cup of liquid skimmed milk. Compensate by reducing consumption of liquid milk.

Use as you please, within reasonable bounds:

Salt substitute
Sugar substitutes (saccharin)—except during first five
    months of pregnancy
Clear broth (not bouillon cubes)
Unsweetened whole gelatin

Artificially sweetened gelatin
Lemon
Vinegar
All spices
All herbs
Sugar-free soft drinks (not cola types)—not more than 8 oz. daily
Coffee free of caffeine (Sanka, Decaf)
Desserts from approved ones mentioned later

Avoid like the plague:

Butter
Sugar-sweetened soft drinks
Sugar-sweetened juices, canned, and frozen fruits
Vegetables packed in sugar-sweetened liquid or sauce (You must read labels carefully!)
Sugar (regardless of its color)
Molasses
Honey
Cookies, cakes, crackers, pretzels, popcorn, potato chips, and all starch-sugar snack foods

Recommended vegetables and fruits follow:

FRUITS	AMOUNT IN ONE SERVING
Apple	1 small (2-inch diameter)
Applesauce	½ cup (no added sugar)
Apricots, fresh	2 medium
Apricots, dried	4 halves
Banana	½ small
Blackberries	1 cup
Blueberries	⅔ cup
Cantaloupe	¼ (6-inch diameter)
Cherries	10 large
Cranberries	1 cup
Dates	2
Figs, fresh	2 large
Figs, dried	1 small

FRUITS	AMOUNT IN ONE SERVING
Grapefruit	½ small
Grapefruit juice	½ cup
Grapes	12 large
Grape juice	¼ cup
Honeydew Melon	⅛ medium
Mango	1 small
Nectarine	1 medium
Orange	1 small
Orange juice	½ cup
Papaya	⅓ medium
Peach	1 medium
Pear	1 small
Persimmon	½ small
Pineapple	½ cup
Pineapple juice	⅓ cup
Plums	2 medium
Prunes, dried	2 medium
Raspberries	1 cup
Rhubarb	1 cup
Strawberries	1 cup
Tangerine	1 cup
Watermelon	1 cup

Be warned that frozen fruits often yield more calories from sugar than from the fruit itself. Avoid canned fruits packed in syrup, whether light or heavy syrup. Choose the water-packed or artificially sweetened variety.

You *must* consume at least *two* cups of vegetables daily, and you can have as much as *four* cups of vegetables daily, chosen from the following list:

Asparagus	Beet Greens
Avocado	Chard
Broccoli	Collards
Brussels Sprouts	Dandelion
Cabbage	Endive
Celery	Kohlrabi
Chicory	Leeks
Cucumbers	Kale

Eggplant	Mustard
Escarole	Spinach
Green Pepper	Turnip Greens
Lettuce	Green or Wax Beans
Mushrooms	Tomatoes
Radishes	Tomato Juice
Sauerkraut	Summer Squash
String Beans	Watercress

Remember that the frequency of eating is as important as the composition of the meals. Do eat six times daily. If at work, protein tablets or foil-wrapped cheese wedges will bridge emergencies when recommended foods are not available.

If you are overweight, the margarine and salad oil recommended in this diet are absolutely essential for a low carbohydrate diet like this one to cause weight loss. In addition, such fats help better control the blood cholesterol.

Glycerin is recommended in the prebreakfast drink, because it is converted into sugar in the body. The conversion is so slow that it does not stimulate the excessive insulin production that is the principle cause of low blood sugar.

While no one vegetable should be overeaten, avocado may receive more emphasis in the diet. This vegetable contains a type of sugar that actually depresses insulin production. Avocado is also rich in unsaturated fat, helpful as noted above to those who are trying to control weight.

Note for those who need guidance in selecting proteins: all animal proteins are roughly equivalent, and therefore are interchangeable when the menu calls for protein. You may exchange meat, fish, fowl, cheeses, milk, and eggs for each other. Consider a glass of milk to be roughly equal to an egg; an ounce of cheese to be equivalent to an ounce of any other animal protein (listed above); two eggs to be roughly equivalent to a four-ounce portion of meat, fish, or fowl. Soy protein is *not* fully equivalent to animal protein, but is useful as a supplement to it *if* served at the same meal.

Though it may have required years of stress and improper diet to ignite your hypoglycemia and its troubles, human nature will seek a one-week cure. This being a disorder for which there is no magic pill, your recovery will take time. While some patients show remarkable improvements in a few weeks, others may need as much as three or four months. If improvement lags at that point, your doctor will explore other possible treatments. The selection of these will be based on considerations not apparent to you. To give you a classic example: there are patients who show a dramatic improvement with the diet and the supplements, but are left with a residual symptom—say, impotence in the male, frigidity in the female. Like most of the symptoms caused by hypoglycemia, these are usually considered psychological in origin, and yet they are often part of the hypoglycemia syndrome, and they are often resistant to the dietary treatment, and they are often conquered when injections of adrenal cortex are added to the regimen.

Human nature still being what it is, as soon as you feel better you will want to know when you can begin to cheat on the diet. Sensibly, never, for hypoglycemia is arrested or controlled; it isn't cured. Actually, some hypoglycemics *are* able to relax the rigors of the diet a bit, at least for an occasional binge with a bit of cake or a small portion of ice cream. Which, of course, ignores the real question: why would you want to return to a form of attenuated gastronomic suicide, with all its potential penalties, just to cater to the pleasures of a degenerated palate?

·2·

The Why and How of Testing and Treatment for the Schizophrenias

PSYCHIATRY HAS DEVELOPED a number of tests which measure the presence and the intensity of symptoms of schizophrenias and other psychoses. Among the better known are the Hoffer-Osmund and the Experiential World Inventory, and there are many others. Their usefulness goes beyond their service in identifying symptoms of a schizophrenia, depression, or dysperceptions. They also serve when properly employed as a sensitive measure of the patient's response to therapy. This is critically important, for these tests may show improvement not visible to the clinical eye, and thereby encourage continuation of a treatment which otherwise might be discarded prematurely. They also sift out the suppression of overt symptoms by the psychotropic drugs, which gives the illusion (again to the clinical eye) that the patient has basically improved, but leaves him still sick, as against the symptomatic improvement with orthomolecular treatment, which nearly always reflects a real alteration in the patient's mental and emotional functioning. Many of these tests are simple true-false or multiple response examinations; others require more effort by the patient, and much more of the practitioner's time in interpretation. All are useful if the patient isn't too withdrawn or confused to cooperate.

Chemical testing in schizophrenia is complex, varying according to the type of sickness involved in this embracive title. In the Sara syndrome, the physician will follow the guidance provided by Pfeiffer's research, who characterizes these patients as having a stress-induced psychosis, accompanied by neurological symptoms, including convulsive episodes; plus abdominal pain, white marks on the nails and stretch marks on the skin; an inability to remember dreams; and a tendency, if Vitamin B_6 doses are too high for this type of patient, to dream excessively. The complexion is China-doll or sallow, and the patient often complains of intolerance to sunlight, with inability to tan, and itching on slight exposure. This is fascinating, since Vitamin B_6 is an important part of the treatment for the Sara syndrome, and this vitamin was recommended more than twenty years ago as a treatment for solar sensitivity (excessive reactions to slight exposure to sunlight). The Sara syndrome, which is defined as a stress-induced Vitamin B_6 and zinc deficiency, is also characterized by inability to eat breakfast, distortions of perception, amnesia, tremor, shaking and muscle spasms, and is often embellished with irregular menstrual periods or cessation of the menses, unexplained fever and chills, anemia which responds only to Vitamin B_6 and a high urinary excretion of kryptopyrrole (above 20 mcg. percent per hundred of urine—this being an alien substance in the blood and urine, which has the capacity to "bind" B_6 and zinc, thereby allowing the patient to suffer deficiency effects while there may be an adequate (but unavailable) amount of the nutrients in the blood.) The kryptopyrrole, which, fascinatingly, is somewhat related to hemoglobin, chlorophyll, and Vitamin B_{12}, has been charged with an hallucinogenic effect, which defines its role in causing some of the problems of perception in schizophrenias. The symptoms just listed need not, of course, be all present simultaneously in a given patient, but when enough of them appear, the psychiatrist may well decide to give large doses of Vitamin B_6—from 1,000 to 2,000 mgs. daily, and an average dose of 80 mgs. of zinc per day. Unlike the psychotropic drug therapies, this treatment presents no discernible risks of any nature—except one which proves its worth: in patients who have responded to the treatment, it must not be discontinued abruptly, for whatever unlikely reason; for such a quick termination of the therapy may bring catatonia or other severe symptoms. Sara syndrome patients who respond to Vitamin B_6 and zinc may secure additional help from supplements of manganese—3 to 5 mgs. daily. Nutritionists will often prefer to use these metals in the chelated form, for better absorption.

It should clearly be understood by the untrained reader that other treatments may be added, for increased benefit. As an example, many of the schizophrenias, including the Sara syndrome group, are marked by excessive copper or lead in the blood and urine. The supplements of zinc may help to bring down the copper levels, necessary because copper is toxic to the nervous system; and supplements of calcium may help to reduce the lead levels, equally neurotoxic, but if the problem is aggravated, the physician may wish to prescribe chelating agents, such as penicillamine or other drugs, more rapidly to reduce the body load of these metals. It must also be remembered that medications, in the right amounts and at the right times, have their place in the orthomolecular scheme, if only to help to bridge difficult periods for the patient. By the same token, large intake of Vitamin B_6, zinc, and manganese may offset the tendency of the blood kryptopyrrole to make these nutrients unavailable to the body, but there are also ways—with niacinamide, for instance—to *reduce* the production of this alien chemical by the body. The point I am making is simple and yet urgent: while nutritional therapies have been administered by everyone from mothers despairing of obtaining professional supervision from cynical or resistant physicians, to social workers and ministers, it's nonetheless true that the trained orthomolecular practitioner may recognize the opportunity for greater or quicker benefits or both, by prescribing additional therapies, many of them unknown to the public, some of them needing prescriptions, a few of them demanding close monitoring of the patient's responses. A good example is lithium therapy, very useful in the treatment of manic-depressives, but requiring skilled hands, for the effective dose varies from patient to patient, the blood levels in response to a given dose similarly vary, and the effective blood level may be very close to the toxic amount.

In childhood schizophrenia and autism, and in hyperactivity and learning difficulties, orthomolecular psychiatrists are administering one to two grams of niacin or niacinamide daily, the dose depending upon body weight; ascorbic acid, one to two grams daily; Vitamin B_6, 200 to 400 mgs. daily, and calcium pantothenate, 400 to 600 mgs. These are starting doses for a child weighing over thirty-five pounds, and the doses of niacin and C are cut in half if the child weighs less. If the child weighs forty-five pounds or more, the practitioner may try to achieve a daily maintenance level of three grams of niacin (or the amide) and three grams of Vitamin C. Side effects are controlled by lowering the dose, and usually come from the niacin. If administered in the form of niacin, rather than the amide, the vitamin produces a feeling of heat and a flushing, for the first five or six doses. This flushing, which is harmless (and more pronounced in redheads) comes from the histamine released in the body as a result of the niacin dosage, and usually subsides as the histamine reserves of the body are exhausted. This produces a side-dividend; severe allergic reactions are less likely when histamine levels are down—you will recall that *anti*histamines are used to treat symptoms of allergy. Despite the flushing action of niacin, the practitioner may specify this form of the vitamin, for the niacinamide form occasionally produces nausea. Some doctors will prescribe niacinamide up to the two-gram level daily, which usually will avoid the nausea, and use niacin for the remaining dosage, which, of course, minimizes the flushing. The two factors—niacin and niacinamide—have the same vitamin action, but differ in other ways. They are interchangeable, obviously, when used in orthomolecular treatment of schizophrenias, emotional disorders, metabolic dysperceptions, and learning disorders. In metabolic dysperception in children, as you realize after reading the story of the ''sad little boy,'' 500 mgs. of niacinamide daily, as the sole nutritional weapon, may restore normal perception.*

Occasionally, large doses of ascorbic acid (Vitamin C) may produce diarrhea or urinary frequency. This is controlled by lowering the dose or, if the given dose is needed, by shifting to another form of the vitamin—sodium ascorbate. Other nutrients are employed: riboflavin, thiamin, Vitamin C, Vitamin E, folic acid, pangamic acid (Vitamin B_{15}), Vitamin B_{12}, and Deaner. The latter is a modified form of choline, which is a B-complex vitamin, so chemically manipulated that it more easily penetrates the barrier guarding the brain. It exercises a stimulating effect on the synthesis by the brain of a neural chemical—acetylcholine—which is vital to the initiation of the nerve impulses conveyed by the brain and nervous systems. Pantothenic acid, another B-complex vitamin, and small amounts of manganese are used with Deaner, to help form that compound. (The physician would phrase it differently: the acetylation of choline depends on pantothenic acid and on a substrate supply of manganese.) Here you see favorable alteration of the chemistry of thinking intelligently invoked by the orthomolecular physician. (And here you will encounter an uninspired objection by the non-orthomolecular practitioner: why give choline, pantothenic acid, and manganese when you don't know if the patient is deficient in them? To which the answer is another question: have you ever found a patient deficient in amphetamine, thorazene, or any of the tranquilizers and psychoenergizers?)

Since the child shares with adults the risk of copper toxicity** or neurologically undesirable high blood levels of

*As this book went to press, I received reports from some orthomolecular psychiatrists who have been achieving excellent responses to very low doses of vitamins and minerals when given in the form of concentrates from natural (food) sources. Such concentrates offer these nutrients in the company of other (trace) substances normally accompanying them in foods. It is scientifically possible that Nature knows—and we do not yet know—how to create "fellow-travelers" which vastly increase the effectiveness of essential nutrients. That is why vitamin supplements are never used as a license for poor dietary habits; they *are* supplements, not substitutes.

**Excessive copper intake may accrue from a combination of a soft water lead, protective mineral supplements are formulated for children, too—zinc, manganese, chromium, calcium, iron, and others, in liquid form, to spare the small child the struggle of swallowing pills and capsules. (Difficulty in swallowing is sometimes one of the symptoms of schizophrenia.) The vitamins are available in solution, too. There are pharmacies specializing in supplying liquid as well as capsulated or tableted vitamin-mineral preparations. They also make the minerals available chelated, for better absorption.

Identification of Vitamin E as a "sex vitamin"—a nomenclature which is redolent of ignorance—has obscured the several actions of the vitamin which make it useful in helping the schizophrenic, the autistic, the hyperactive, and the sufferer with a learning disability. The vitamin dampens the transmission of anxiety impulses from the diencephalon to the cortex, which translates it as a natural, harmless, tranquilizing nutrient. It is also involved in the chemistries of RNA and DNA, and in those of the ubiquinones; these actions make it fundamental to the basic chemistry of the cell, and to the forces of energy metabolism in cell and body. It is also a potent and harmless antioxidant, a consideration of importance in those diseases, like schizophrenia, where oxidation of chemicals normal to the body, it has been postulated, may result in formation of alien and hallucinogenic reaction products. Finally, Vitamin E is known to block the action of porphyrin, a substance related to the kryptopyrrole previously discussed, and which is known to contribute to a type of psychosis. However, these multiple actions are achieved only if the vitamin is employed in the proper form. This is not "alpha-tocopherol" or any other variation of this single form of the vitamin. The complete actions are obtained only from a combination of all the forms of Vitamin E, which translates into "mixed tocopherols." This represents alpha,

---

supply and copper piping. It is a wise precaution to discard the "standing water" in the pipeline, by letting the water run for four or five minutes before drawing it for morning beverages, dilution of fruit juices, etc.

beta, gamma, and delta tocopherols. The label may properly state that the activity is measured in terms of the alpha, but must also state that "mixed tocopherols" are present.* The dosage used, measured in terms of the alpha potency, may go up to 1,600 units daily, for an adult. Small children may be given 50 to 100 mgs. daily.

Under such a therapeutic regime, results may take two to six months before gains become unmistakable, though they are sometimes dramatically quick. Concentration and the memory span improve, hyperactivity diminishes; in the schizophrenic child, dysperceptions become less pronounced or disappear, and the child is no longer a mercurial irritant to his parents, teachers, and schoolmates.

Cott notes as an observation particularly important to parents of children with learning difficulties that learning-disabled children tend to share a group of characteristics which will be interesting to the reader who has carefully studied the preceding discussions of hypoglycemia. He finds that these children have a high incidence of low blood sugar and food allergies, and that there is an abnormally high history of diabetes in the families of this group. Not by coincidence, he emphasizes that the dietary habits of these children lean toward cereals, sweets, and foods prepared with sugar—the very selections they should be minimizing or avoiding. (These remarks would, of course, apply also to schizophrenic children, many of whom are hypoglycemic; all the more because, as it was previously noted, there is evidence that wheat may be severely disturbing to the schizophrenic.)

Contrary to the establishment's picture of the orthomolecular psychiatrist and pediatrician as a practitioner obsessed with a monomania in therapy—only the use of vitamins, minerals, and controlled diet—Cott emphasizes that perceptual-motor techniques should be employed in disturbed and

---

*The beta, gamma, and delta forms of the vitamin have great antioxidant activity, but virtually no effect on the chemistry of the cell. The alpha form has very little antioxidant effect, but profound action on cell chemistry.

learning-disabled children while efforts to "balance" them biochemically are in progress.

We have not exhausted the nutritional substances on which orthomolecular therapies may draw. Nucleic acid involved in the transmission of genetic instructions to the molecules of life, may be administered in the form of a supplement. In the brain-injured child or adult, a 27-carbon waxy long-chain alcohol, derived from wheat germ oil, shows promise in stimulating a process neurologists are taught can't be stimulated: repair of damaged brain nerve cells. Since folic acid and Vitamin B_{12} work with Vitamin B_6, they are frequently given together. Such interrelationships and certain antagonisms among nutrients motivate the practitioner in his recommendations. Doses of zinc may reduce elevated blood copper and increase copper excretion, which in schizophrenics is often low. However, it mustn't be thought that copper is *always* a villain; depression may be caused by a copper overload, which sometimes is responsible for premenstrual "lows" even in normal women; but depression has been treated successfully *with* copper, when blood levels were abnormally low. (Don't complain about the complexities of the orthomolecular: it's *you* who are complex.) Elevation of lead in the blood is sometimes lessened with calcium, but the mineral and zinc are also antagonistic, and doses of the two must be balanced. Vitamin B_6 deficiency, contrary to the statements of some of the orthomolecular authorities, may be induced by high dosage of niacin in some (not all) patients, requiring use of both vitamins, simultaneously, even when the Sara syndrome is not the problem.

In the treatment of schizophrenias in the older child and the adult, the authorities mold the therapy in accordance with the duration and the severity of the sickness. In early, mild schizophrenia, doses of niacin or niacinamide alone or with Vitamin B_6 may (and often do) prove the key to the door of recovery. A mild dose of a mild tranquilizer may also be needed—mild because the vitamin therapy often sharply increases the effectiveness of the tranquilizer action. Approximately three to twelve grams of niacin or niacinamide, or a combination of the two, may be used.* It should be emphasized that only very early, quite mild schizophrenias are susceptible to this beginning phase therapy, which, as I explained earlier, explains why it *had* to fail when applied to a hospital population which could have represented no mild and no early cases; yet this "study" is often cited as "proof" of the invalidity of orthomolecular claims.

In some cases, large doses of Vitamin C will be used—as high as 60 grams per day, and probably not less than one or two grams. In part, the justification for this treatment is based on the observation that schizophrenics tend to retain a much larger percentage of these large doses than normals do; the retention is gradually reduced as the schizophrenic begins to recover. This is taken as an indication that while he is sick, the vitamin is critically needed to help him to "detoxify" his system; and in recovery, the detoxification has been accomplished, the need for the vitamin correspondingly reduced, and the excretion, as a corollary, increased.

These older schizophrenics may also receive supplements of Vitamin E. If hypoglycemic, they will be placed on the appropriate diet. If allergic, the offending foods and factors will be removed from the external and internal environments.

If these measures are unsuccessful or the improvement strikes a plateau, ECT may be used—electro-convulsive therapy. I have always regarded this as an atavistic reflection of the ancient snake pit, used then in the hope that fright might scare the demons out of the body; but at the present state of the imperfect art, ECT sometimes means the difference between full response and partial, or partial response and none. If there is distinct improvement which is held for a week or so after the last treatment, and the vitamin therapy is continued, there is then hope that the improvement will be main-

---

*Niacin is an acid (its other name is nicotinic acid), and in those subject to hyperacidity of the stomach, may cause heartburn. The physician may prevent this by dissolving the vitamin dose in water and adding bicarbonate of soda, very gradually, until the solution stops fizzing, which means the acid is neutralized. Iced, this drink is tasteless and odorless, and will no longer cause indigestion even in the susceptible.

tained. ECT may be applied on one side of the brain or on both—the choice dictated by the severity of the sickness. In a very mild but persistent illness, the ECT might be employed only on the non-dominant side of the brain, offering the advantage that the posttreatment confusion and transient loss of memory will be mild. Bilateral ECT may cause greater confusion and amnesia, but with the orthomolecular therapy preceding and following it, these, too, pass.

In chronic cases of severe schizophrenia, doses of the vitamins will be increased, more potent tranquilizers employed, measures taken against excessive copper and lead; and with all the other modalities—elimination of allergens, etc.—this group will, of course, have the least optimistic prognosis. Nonetheless, let me emphasize that even some of these patients come back to social and vocational usefulness. To put it all into simple arithmetic: if the orthomolecular therapist is working with a mixed population which has the ''normal'' distribution of patients—from early, mild cases to extremely severe, chronic ones—his overall percentage of success should approximate 80 percent. And when you consider the entities of disease he is challenging—the alcoholic, the schizophrenic, the manic-depressive, the autistic, the brain-damaged, the retarded, the hyperactive, and the ''learning problem''—one must in fairness remember the old English proverb: ''If every man would mend a man, then would all men be mended.'' The orthomolecular practitioner mends his man, and more.

We've learned that the glucose tolerance test, over a six-hour period, is a reasonably accurate way of identifying hypoglycemia. With the addition of stress during the fourth and fifth-hour periods, the test becomes more accurate. There are, however, other chemistries the physician may explore. One of these is salt metabolism, which will tend to be disturbed in those patients with low blood sugar who do not respond to the hypoglycemia diet alone, but require treatment with adrenal cortical hormones. If the physician doesn't wish to wait for four or six weeks, to see what response there is to the dietary-and-vitamin-mineral therapy, he can do a "salt-dumping" test to identify adrenal insufficiency. He will ask for a twenty-four-hour urine, which will be analyzed for sodium, potassium, and chloride. For the second urine test, you will be asked to consume about the same amount of food, in a day's period, and then to swallow 10 grams of salt in water, in a half hour. The twenty-four-hour-urine is collected, and analyzed for sodium, potassium, and choloride. If there is any appreciable difference in the levels, the physician will tell you that you are "dumping salt," which in turn is taken as evidence that certain hormones are not being produced adequately by the adrenal cortex. This, of course, would then justify adding doses of adrenal cortex hormones to your treatment, given either by injection or, infrequently, in the oral form (adrenal protomorphogens in tablet form).

If the physician gives you a test for the blood level of Nicotinamide Adenine Dinucleotide, he is simultaneously learning three important facts about your personal chemistry. First, whether you're deficient in this compound, which would mean deficiency in niacin. Second, this test tells him whether you have the chemistry characteristic of a schizophrenia, though it doesn't necessarily mean that you have that disorder. Third, when your supply of this compound is low, it means that hypoglycemia can be anticipated, since NAD is vital in control over the metabolism of starches and sugars. A blood sample for NAD testing is taken before the glucose tolerance test starts, and another is taken at the fourth hour of the test, which is the period when the NAD level is likely to be lowest. The NAD levels are used as a guide in megavitamin doses of niacin.

A fascinating substance vital to energy processes is adenosine triphosphate. This is the energy-laden compound which makes possible the cold light of the firefly, and it is responsible for the phenomenon of the chicken which continues to run after it has been decapitated—so much energy still being derived from the adenosine compound. It is made from essential amino acids, B complex vitamins, and phospholipids (phosphorus combined chemically with fats), catalyzed by magnesium. Deficiencies in all these factors are easily possible in the sugar-laden diet that helps to initiate low blood sugar; and it follows that hypoglycemics tend to be low in ATP. This compound also can increase the efficiency of adrenal cortical functions, as improved adrenal function can increase the production of ATP. Sodium and potassium are needed for ideal production of ATP; this explains why it is important to learn if you are "dumping salt." One method of helping to raise adenosine triphosphate production is by supplementary intake of adenosine-5-monophosphate, which is one of the building blocks from which the body makes ATP. (The preliminary form of the compound is available in tablets which are absorbed by placing them under the tongue.) A fasting blood sample and a four-hour sample of blood, drawn during the glucose tolerance test, are used for determination of ATP levels. This is an important test for hypoglycemics, since deficiency in the factor means that you can't adequately create energy from carbohydrates, and explains some of the weakness hypoglycemics suffer.

Both a contributor to the troubles of the hypoglycemic, and a result of the diet eaten by those who ultimately become hypoglycemic, is underactivity of the thyroid gland. Elaborate and sensitive tests for the function of this gland are available, but your physician, in place of the PBI, the T3, and the T4 tests, may choose a much simpler, less expensive, and surprisingly accurate method. He will instruct you, on awakening, to place a thermometer in the armpit and keep it there for ten minutes. A temperature of less than 97.8° will indicate an underactive thyroid gland. This uncomplicated procedure is frequently a more sensitive index of your need for thyroid than the more elaborate and costly laboratory methods. In fact, when the laboratory denies your need for extra thyroid, but the underarm test insists you do need it, the physician's experience may tell him you may indeed profit by thyroid medication, and the dividends may include reduction of blood cholesterol, more energy, fewer colds, less constipation, better growth of nails and hair, and beneficial changes in personality. With the thyroid supplement, the doctor may give you extra thiamin (Vitamin B_1), iodine, and a diet free of such antithyroid foods as liver, the cabbage family, soy products, and those high in carotene. These dietary taboos are operative only when there is a family history of goiter, or your thyroid deficiency is pronounced.

A complete blood chemistry, a "CBC" will be ordered.* You will be given the mauve test, which identifies the troublemaking factor (kryptopyrrole) you encountered in the history of Sara, and which is part of the problem of some schizophrenics. Tests aimed at nutritional deficiency will include determinations of serum Vitamin B_{12}, magnesium, calcium (both total and unbound), the Figlu test for folic acid levels, pyruvic acid (for thiamin deficiency), and galactose tolerance. The latter is a form of milk sugar, lactose, to which some people show an intolerance which will create a type of hypoglycemia. Many of these tests are especially important to schizophrenics; some are for hypoglycemics; others bear upon problems of the emotionally disturbed, the retarded, and the autistic; and all of the tests will be needed by some patients. Hair tests for minerals may be made. The choice of hair as a testing medium is based on the fact that the blood chemistries change kaleidoscopically, from day to day, while the hair values give a more stable view of the overall mineral nutrition. Your physician will discuss with you the problems created by hair dyes, shampoos, and conditioners, some of which will throw the test values off. A few of such products, for instance, will raise the lead content of the hair to a level which would be alarming, if it really reflected what's in the body.

The time at which a test is given is critical, as you realize from the prior observations of the differences in glucose tol-

---

*Research into the chemistry of schizophrenia has resulted in stress on the importance of certain biochemical tests which were previously of little interest to the physician, and none to the psychiatrist. Methylated and substituted spermine and spermidines are examples. When the orthomolecular physician asks for tests of levels of these factors, it's because Pfeiffer and his coworkers have linked a high level of spermidine with abnormal thinking and dysperception of time in the schizophrenic.

erance shown by an early morning test as compared with one which runs into the afternoon. It will be of interest to schizophrenics that the Hoffer-Osmund test for schizophrenia may give quite different results when administered in the first hour of a glucose tolerance test, when the blood sugar levels will ordinarily be up, as compared with the results in the fourth hour. Administration of the test is justified, if the patient is not too confused to understand it, because it not only is helpful as a diagnostic tool to identify schizophrenia, but it also helps to differentiate the schizophrenic from the neurotic and from the patient with a personality disorder. This differentiation is important, since the schizophrenic needs more intensive treatment. The reactions during the glucose tolerance tests themselves help to differentiate: the hypoglycemic who is not schizophrenic may have some perceptual distortions and feel more depressed; the schizophrenic is very likely to show specific evidence of his disorder, particularly if stressed while the test is under way.

Perhaps most puzzling to the patient of all the physician's decisions is the one which leads him to prescribe extra intake of a vitamin or other nutrient for which the patient, on the basis of the blood testing, has no need. But we have no tests for *need;* we can only test for what's *there*. A reading at the lower end of the normal range may not be normal for you, and far less than optimal. Which differs not at all from the physician's practice with doses of thyroid hormone: many a patient has been protected against a heart attack by supplements of thyroid hormone which, according to the chemical tests, weren't critically needed. So it is that extra Vitamin B_{12}, given to patients whose blood tests showed no deficiency, has rescued some of them from paranoid psychoses or from perceptual distortion. Or extra Vitamin B_1, again unneeded in the light of the blood tests, has helped some patients to throw off some part of their depression. Or extra niacinamide, also not needed on the basis of the blood test, has brought clarity to confused thinking. Because, you see, not only does the blood level say nothing about your need, but it offers no guarantee that what is there is necessarily efficiently reaching the tissues. Metabolic errors in enzyme chemistries may throw up a partial block; transport failures in the body do occur; maladaptive reactions may negate the usefulness of the nutrient. All this doesn't make the testing academic. It serves as a guide, however rough, in the tangled chemistries of the complex organism we inhabit.

·3·

The Why and How of Testing and Treatment for Psychoallergy

ALLERGIES WHICH STRIKE like malign arrows directly at the brain and nervous system, with formidable influence on the patient's perceptions of reality, have been demonstrated in thousands of patients, and are known to play a significant role in complicating the perceptual distortions of schizophrenics. Like the hypoglycemias, psychoallergies are often undetected because the symptoms so faithfully resemble those of psychosis or neurosis, or because they are so subjective, or because the medical man will not find what he is not seeking. It is entirely possible, emphasizes Dr. Marshall Mandell, pioneer neuroallergist, that mental patients in institutions are being fed the very foods which touch off cerebral allergies and which, thereby, are helping to keep them sick.

It is appallingly easy to mistake the symptoms of psychoallergy for those of a severe neurosis. Marked changes in body and brain chemistry and in the permeability of cell membranes are caused by allergy. It is no more strange that an allergic reaction may cause depression than it is inconceivable that an hallucinogenic chemical, produced within the body, could cause a little boy to receive visits from his dead grandfather, appearing in the shape of a purple ball—a phenomenon relieved by megavitamin therapy, exactly as allergic reactions in the brain are cancelled by doses of Vitamin B_6 and Vitamin C.

Wheat, corn, milk, tobacco, products derived from petroleum, insecticides, and many other environmental substances to which we are all exposed, have been shown—both in well people and in schizophrenics—to cause grossly psychotic reactions. The symptoms have ranged from weakness, dizziness, anxiety, and depression, to major psychotic episodes, including catatonia, megalomania, visual and auditory hallucinations, and serious attempts at suicide. Some patients react to different foods or chemicals with similar symptoms, but in others, each food produces a different reaction, often in different organs of the body. To add to the complexity of these responses, exposure to an allergen may trigger *learned* behavior, as was previously pointed out. Thus a patient might feel great hostility toward a relative for real (or, frequently, imagined) mistreatment. That hostility may be elicited in the same patient by exposure to a food or chemical to which he is markedly allergic.

Though appropriately in the context of this book I have emphasized the emotional and the mental symptoms that allergy may cause, it should be remembered that physical symptoms may result, too, and may be severe, including headaches, dizziness, sleepiness, insomnia, changes in the heart rate (up or down), extra systoles, indigestion, heartburn, diarrhea, constipation, tension, weakness, elevation or lowering of blood pressure, hives, psoriasis, and colitis. In children, untreated allergy may contribute to marked learning difficulties, convulsive disorders, susceptibility to respiratory infections, irritability, and constant fatigue—part of what Dr. Ray Wunderlich, specialist in children's allergic problems, calls the neuroallergic syndrome. In autistic children, removal of allergens from the diet has been helpful, just as some autistic children have responded favorably to megavitamin treatment.

Grouped under the term ''neuroallergic reactions'' are a number of abnormal processes. Some patients who suffer from them are chemically defective organisms requiring special protection against the threats of an environment laden with chemicals, food additives, and allergenic foods and beverages. The responses to the allergy tests may reflect genuine allergy—whatever that may be, there being differences of professional opinion—or nutritional deficiency, or an error of body chemistry which makes a common substance, well tolerated by most of us, toxic. So it is that a positive reaction to an allergy test tells the doctor you're reacting, but patient investigation, with your full cooperation, will be needed to determine *why*. Meanwhile, the physician will try to give you relief by any one of a number of methods. Nutritional deficiencies will be corrected, both with foods and supplements, but in the choice of the supplements, the medical man will prefer those made with no fillers or as little of these as possible, for each such addition to your intake brings up the possibility of reaction in a sensitive patient. Offending substances, where possible, will be excluded from your external and internal environments, including everything from foods to molds to automobile exhaust and other hydrocarbons. If petrochemicals turn out to be a nemesis of yours, you will be instructed not to use pens based on petroleum byproducts, or kitchen cleaners containing them; and you may even have to change the heating source in your home, for an oil burner can cause great trouble for those very sensitive to petroleum hydrocarbons. Antidotal doses of Vitamin C and Vitamin B_6 may be ordered to offset the allergic reactions which evade the doctor's shield of protection for you, or he may prescribe doses of sodium and potassium bicarbonate or order inhalation of carbon dioxide, to change the acid-alkaline balance of your blood. If the disturbing substance is unavoidable, the physician may try to desensitize you, in the fashion in which allergists traditionally have immunized patients, by small and gradually increasing injections of the factor.

A little realized source of difficulty derives from the addictiveness of foods to which you are allergic. Those you *deeply* crave are likely to be the foods causing or aggravating your troubles with hypoglycemia, schizophrenia, and other disorders. The prime reason for addiction rests on the fact that each dose of an offending food serves as a temporary antidote for the disturbing effects of the previous portion. This mechanism isn't yet understood, and the antidotal effect is of course not complete; the residual impact creates the craving for the next portion. For these reasons, as I previously noted, the practitioner will ask you to keep a diary of your intake of foods, beverages, and medications, with a complete list of any discernible reactions, no matter how subjective. He will want to know where you went, what you did, what made you feel good or better, what made you feel worse or ill. This information will then serve as a background against which he will measure your test reactions to foods, chemicals, fumes, additives, beverages, tobacco, etc. Some tests he may ask you to do at home—such as sniffing a little fresh paint, or inhaling the vapor of a marker pen, or exposing yourself briefly to cats, dogs, dust, and pollens. Some will be done by the sublingual (under the tongue) test previously described, which must be medically supervised.

Since the foods to which the patient is allergic are often those to which he becomes addicted and repeats most often, the physician may prescribe a rotated diet. Some doctors use a four-day rotation; some extend it to a week. The menu plan for a four-day rotation might specify beef on Monday, which would mean that the entrée at *all* meals, that day, would be a beef dish, sans seasoning or other additions. Oranges and apples would be the only fruits that day. The vegetables might include several varieties of squash, plus lettuce. The starch might be derived from baked potato. Wheat would not be permitted, milk eliminated on that day, and eggs are verboten. On Tuesday, the protein dish—for all meals—would be some kind of fish. Sweet potatoes would be the starch. Tangerines or bananas might be the fruit, and so on. You gather that the menus are monotonous, and so they are, but the ordeal is worthwhile if it helps to relieve perceptual distortion, or aids a schizophrenic, or improves an autistic child, or is helpful in relieving a member of the family from such possible penalties for allergy as headache, postnasal drip, stomach ache, mental sluggishness, fatigue, and irritability.*

*An excellent brief presentation of a pair of rotation diets is available to your physician by consulting the *Journal of Orthomolecular Psychiatry,*

It must be remembered that the troublemaking substances in the diet need not be directly from the food or beverages. The chemicals used in can linings are sometimes offenders. Plastic wrapping allows plasticizer to be picked up by the protein or fat of the food. Water known to be free of contaminants may relieve some patients of symptoms caused by the bizarre array of chemicals coming to us from "potable" drinking water in many cities. If insecticide residues are touching off reactions, it will be necessary to find a trustworthy source of unsprayed foods, and meat from animals not subjected to these toxic substances in *their* environment and *their* food. (I recall a patient with severe inflammation of the pancreas who found relief from her frequent attacks by shifting to organically grown food, but she found it necessary to have it tested, for some sources proved to be unreliable.)

As testing for allergies by diet rotation progresses, and offending foods and beverages are deleted, it becomes possible for the physician to add new items to be evaluated, which ultimately may allow considerable broadening of the menus. Restoration of allergic foods to the diet, though, is unwise, for their effects may seem innocuous, but can prove to be additive, finally exploding in a full-fledged outbreak of the original symptoms of allergy. A very occasional indulgence in a large portion of an offending food is usually safer than every day consumption of small amounts; but Rees recommends neither procedure.

The mother faced with the rotation menu may wonder if recovery of the patient at the expense of a nervous breakdown for the cook, faced with adding these menus to those of the family, is worthwhile. The obvious answer is to place the entire family on the rotation diet. Properly planned, it can be

---

Vol. 2, No. 3, page 93, in an article by Dr. Elizabeth Lodge Rees. Where allergies are severe and multiple, and more complete guidance is needed, there is an excellent book published by the New England Foundation of Allergic and Environmental Diseases, 3 Brush Street, Norwalk, Connecticut 06850. It is titled *Management of Complex Allergies—the Patient's Guide*, by Natalie Golos.

perfectly good nutrition, and if the patient is truly being made ill—or more ill—by uncontrolled allergies, the sacrifice will not long be considered such, as the sufferer improves. Moreover, if the patient is a child and allergic, there is a good chance that other members of the family share the tendency, which means that they, too, benefit by the procedure.

When you visit a neurological allergist or a psychiatrist practicing in that field, it will save time if you are armed with a diary which relates symptoms to food intake. The diary should give the day and the exact time of taking each food, snack, or beverage, with some idea of sizes or portions. It should describe all symptoms occurring during the night, and any physical or mental symptoms occurring after arising. It should list everything eaten for breakfast, and any symptoms that follow breakfast—with careful notes of the times at which the symptoms appeared. The diary must list all snacks, and describe and give the time of symptoms following these. The same is done with the noon meal—content, and following symptoms, with time of occurrence; and so with afternoon snacks, evening meal, and so on. If you are exposed during the day to animals or molds, pollens, chemical fumes, smoke, odors, or dust—any of these in unusual amounts—that should be recorded, and any following symptoms. The diary should describe where you went, what you did, anything you did that made you feel good, anything that created symptoms. A week before visiting the physician, begin the diary. It will help the practitioner to help you, in more ways than you now know. Food testing, for instance, can be done only on foods that have been eaten three times a week or more. The medical man will tell you that foods that have not been eaten frequently must be taken daily for at least one week before he makes the test.

Complex, you think? Not so complex as trying to live with a hyperactive child. Not so complex nor so painful as watching someone you love struggling with twisted thoughts and distorted emotions. In no way as complex and distressing as trying, as a chemically defective person, to think straight and function in a contaminated world.

Finally, those who seek the specialized services of a neuro-allergist should communicate with the Alan Mandell Center of Bio-Ecologic Diseases, 3 Brush St., Norwalk, Connecticut 06850.

Inquiries should *not* be addressed to the author, on whose hapless head now descends a volume of mail—uninvited and beyond management—which no single individual could read, much less answer. Which is not written in an unkindly way. It is sympathy for those who seek and who have been denied that compelled the writing of this book.

·4·

Questions from Patients and Their Families

Q. Can ordinary tap water cause psychiatric symptoms?

A. Both physical and mental disturbances can be caused by the chlorine or other chemicals in tap water. The physical symptoms can include stuffy nose, dryness or soreness of the throat and eyes, tightness of the chest, headaches, and a feeling of inner shakiness. Arthritis has been caused by the chlorine in water, and disappeared when the patient was restricted to a pure spring (mineral) water.

Q. In such problems (as reacting to the chlorination of water) wouldn't it be best to switch to distilled water?

A. Distilled water is mineral-hungry, and will pick up minerals from the body, which then are lost by excretion. A pure mineral water is preferable.

Q. Is there proof that psychotherapy doesn't help schizophrenics?

A. If you're thinking in terms of curing the disease, there is a great deal of proof that psychotherapy does nothing. This includes a study of re-admission rates in a three-year period by schizophrenics who received psychotherapy and a group receiving rou-

tine hospital care. Numerous studies confirm thi
finding. This doesn't mean that schizophrenics ma
not be helped through some of their problems witl
skilled psychotherapy.

Q. Are there specific vitamin deficiencies that ca
cause depression?

A. There is evidence that depression may be one of th
symptoms resulting from pantothenic acid defi
ciency. So with deficiency in riboflavin, thiamin
biotin, and niacin.

Q. In schizophrenic and autistic children, what migh
be some of the early changes indicating a respons
to orthomolecular treatment?

A. Hyperactivity may diminish. The children may be
gin to understand orders. Their ability to commu
nicate, by speech and other means, may improve
Many of them become more affectionate.

Q. I noticed that as my schizophrenic brother re
sponded to the megavitamins and the diet, he be
came noticeably more nervous for the first fev
weeks. Is this an unusual response?

A. In the first four to six weeks of psycho-nutrition, man
schizophrenics do feel more nervous. This is why th
practitioner may for some time continue mild dose
of a tranquilizer.

Q. My physician, in addition to vitamins and mineral
and a hypoglycemia diet, prescribed capsules o
tryptophane, which I understand is an amino aci
which is supplied by protein. I'm eating plenty c
protein foods—why the tryptophane capsules?

A. To give you a quote: those whose diets supply onl
the RDA (recommended dietary allowance) of nu
trients may be mentally deprived, and tryptophan
is a good example. Intake only 30 percent highe

than the RDA has dramatically reduced the number of psychiatric symptoms in some patients. The amino acid in such modest doses has not caused any reported difficulties.

Q. My physician says my anxiety isn't caused by anything in my life or life-style, except my diet. He says I have elevated lactic acid in the blood, but he hasn't prescribed anything to correct this, which he blames for the anxiety. Is there anything that would reduce this lactic acid?

A. A frequent cause of elevated lactic acid in the blood is a calcium deficiency. Correction of that may banish the anxiety. If extra calcium isn't taken, a deficiency in it may be directly caused by the lactic acid, which has the capacity to "bind" the calcium, making it unavailable to the body. This is another example of the fallacy of a blood test: what's there may not always be useful.

Q. When I told my previous psychiatrist that the "voices" caused by my schizophrenia had disappeared within two weeks of my starting treatment with niacinamide, he said he can accomplish the same thing with any one of a dozen tranquilizers. Is this true?

A. For some patients (and some tranquilizers) it is true. The added dividend from the vitamin therapy is not provided by the drugs: not only do the voices disappear in the patient responding to the psycho-nutrition; so does the severity of the schizophrenic symptoms. The tranquilizer may silence the voices, but not silence the schizophrenia itself; and the patient remains then essentially as sick as he was. With psycho-nutrition, the actual score on a test for schizophrenia may drop to normal, as the voices fade out, or come to be viewed for what they are: the patient's own thoughts.

Q. I am a recovered schizophrenic-hypoglycemic. How long must I stay on the hypoglycemia diet?

A. Some patients can cheat a little, at intervals; some never can. Hypoglycemia isn't cured—it's arrested. For most patients, overprocessed sugar and starch in small amounts are like a small dose of carbolic acid.

Q. I was successfully treated for schizophrenia with megavitamins, diet, and a tranquilizer, plus removing some foods to which I'm allergic. Simultaneously, an arthritis I was told I'd have to learn to live with—hypertrophic arthritis—disappeared. Was this coincidence, or was it because I stopped eating sugar and the foods to which I was allergic?

A. The large doses of Vitamin B_6 you took, plus the potassium in your diet, may have been the key to recovery from the arthritis. That type of arthritis, it has been urged by Dr. John Ellis, should be re-labeled for what it is: a product of a specific deficiency in this vitamin and mineral.

Q. My doctor says that because I'm a redhead, he'd rather give me niacinamide than niacin. Can you explain why?

A. Niacin causes flushing, and redheads tend to have more severe flushes, which for some patients prove disturbing.

Q. My hyperactive boy was also a bed-wetter, and that's disappearing as his condition improves. Is there a special nutrient in his vitamin supplements that might be responsible for his learning to control his bladder?

A. Vitamin E has been reported helpful in some cases of bed-wetting. Magnesium also.

Q. Does it make any difference whether the vitamins and minerals are taken before or after a meal?

A. None, in most people. They work with food, and should be taken with it—whether before or after.

Q. Why isn't honey a good substitute for sugar?

A. Ordinary sugar in the body is converted into glucose and fructose (fruit sugar). Research has shown that it is the fruit sugar—of which honey is a *rich* source—that causes most of the trouble blamed on ordinary sugar. Anything adverse caused by large doses of sugar can be caused more intensively and faster by fruit sugar. There is therefore no form of sugar which is good food, and none which is to be preferred by hypoglycemics.

Q. What about artificial sweeteners?

A. Saccharin and cyclamate are still being studied, and no pronouncements have yet been made. The chemist warns us that these are small molecules, and thereby capable of passing barriers in the body which shouldn't be invaded. If you must perpetuate your sweet tooth with artificial sweeteners, you might help protect yourself by stopping their use completely for a full week, every third week, thereby letting the body get rid of the material. The new protein sweetener, not yet marketed, will for most people be a better choice, but must not be used if the physician detects phenylpyruvia in the patient or the family. Get into the habit of tasting beverages before you sweeten them, and cutting down on the absurdly large amount of sugar in most recipes. If done gradually, the change will be imperceptible to the family.

Q. Can severe catatonia be treated successfully the psycho-nutrition way?

A. The very first case to respond to orthomolecular

treatment was that of a man with severe catatonia. He has been well ever since.

Q. Can orthomolecular treatment help a drug addict?
A. Many reports so indicate. This includes not only doses of niacin, Vitamin C, Vitamin B$_6$, and Vitamin E, but a hypoglycemia diet. Some of these addicts are definitely suffering from low blood sugar, for the symptoms of which they find release in drugs.

Q. Has anyone studied the possibility of using psychonutrition for some of the genuinely intelligent students who drop out of high school and college?
A. We believe, though controlled studies have yet to be done, that the functioning of many of these dropouts could be raised to a significantly higher level by nutritional treatment . . . enough of an improvement to stimulate some of them into completing their educations.

Q. My premenstrual week and the first day of menstruation were perfectly awful before I was treated for schizophrenia by a medical nutritionist. Now they're so free of symptoms that I keep holding my breath, thinking the improvement might have been a coincidence. Could it have been?
A. Possibly, but probably not. With improvement of liver function as a result of corrected diet, higher in protein and lower in sugar, plus supplements of the Vitamin B complex, I have reported similar improvements in premenstrual tension, backache, cramps, water retention and weight gain, breast cysts, and premenstrual hysteria and craving for sweets, dizziness, etc., in girls who were not schizophrenic.

Q. If you continue to feel weak, irritable, and nervous on a hypoglycemia diet, and you have no allergies, what's the next step?

A. In some cases, additional allowances of complex carbohydrates, such as baked potato, spaghetti, etc. In a percentage of these cases, it will also be necessary to reduce slightly the overall amount of fat in the diet. Sometimes the addition of half a baked potato, twice daily, proves the key to recovery. This means, of course, that our carbohydrate needs, like all others, differ from person to person; and so will tolerance to a low carbohydrate diet.

Q. My physician is away, and I can't reach him to ask why the lithium he used to overcome my depression seems to have stimulated my appetite. If I start to gain weight, I'll be depressed all over again. What should I do?

A. Thirst and stimulation of appetite are sometimes symptoms of too high a level of lithium in the blood. Any competent physician can order tests to check this, and adjust your dose to keep you out of trouble.

Q. Food used to be tasteless when I was deep in schizophrenia. Now it seems my sense of taste is sharper than it ever was. Did schizophrenia affect that?

A. A zinc deficiency, with or without schizophrenia, can cause loss of both a sense of taste and a sense of smell. Probably your physician gave you zinc, as part of your treatment. In schizophrenia, the sense of taste is more often deranged than completely missing: foods taste terrible to many patients.

Q. My son's tendency to smack up cars has lessened noticeably since he's on niacinamide. Is this coincidence?

A. Schizophrenics very often don't realize that the car they're driving is too close to the one in front, or over the line in the middle of the road. As they recover, these dysperceptions lessen or disappear. This obviously would lead to driving that's more accident-free.

Q. I have the impression that my tendency to stutter is less now, even when I'm under emotional pressure. Could it be because of the megavitamins that this improvement has taken place?

A. I've been trying for years to persuade speech therapists to experiment with megavitamin doses and corrected diets in speech impediments. I have a distinct impression that some stuttering is an audiogenic seizure directly caused by a high and unsatisfied nutritional requirement.

L'Envoi: For Those Who Would Like to Be Better Than "Normal"

You HAVE READ that non-hypoglycemics may feel and function better on a hypoglycemia-type diet, sugar-free, low in carbohydrates, and taken in frequent small meals. You have read of a man whose personality changed dramatically for the better after a relatively small increase in his intake of calcium pantothenate. Described earlier were non-psychotics whose thinking clarified when they were given supplements of niacinamide. Has it occurred to you that we always manage to confuse *average* with *normal,* a semantic trap in which *you* and millions of others may lose an opportunity for nutritional self-improvement?

To escape the trap, you must first realize that an "average nutritional requirement" may be a convenient tool for Washington statisticians, which for *you* may place a nutritional ceiling upon you, an invisible tether which will inescapably restrict your potential. The metaphor is mixed, but you have read this book and thereby surely realize that our biochemical differences are greater than our similarities, and our nutritional needs vary, similarly. *You* may not tolerate a low carbohydrate diet, as there are those who profit on a high-fat, high-cholesterol diet, and those who find it a pathway to trouble. *You,* who gain weight merely by sniffing the aroma of a baking cake, may solve your problem completely by dropping your intake of sugar as low as possible, and holding your intake of carbohydrates (starches) to about 60 grams a day.

You may do well on three meals daily; there are those who feel infinitely better on six. A multiple vitamin, multiple mineral and Vitamin B complex supplement may turn ''sub-oxidizers'' into more vital people, supercharged with a new found initiative and heightened resistance to fatigue and stress. The same supplements may restore a ''lost'' premenstrual week to a productive one, for millions of women. Coupled with a hypoglycemia diet, these supplements may build resistance to allergies. None of the laboratory tests can evaluate the potential you might reach by altering your nutrient intake to fulfill the peculiarly unique requirements of *your* body, *your* metabolism.

This much we can definitely say: research has shown that nutritional requirements in animals of the same genetic strain may vary by a factor of five; occasionally, by a factor of thirty or forty. Those few experiments which have measured the differences in nutritional needs of man have arrived at the same conclusion: they differ by a factor of at least five, and sometimes more. Considering the diversity of man's genetic backgrounds, there would be no excuse for assuming man to be an exception. Therefore, this suggestion: it might be most rewarding to determine if your body and mind have been functioning under handicaps. It is not only possible but it may be probable that nutritional limitations in your childhood are now restricting your potential as an adult. We know that this can happen, and we know that it is frequently reversible. It is possible that your pattern of diet as an adult has not met your optimal needs, and that, too, is remediable. Start by reading texts on nutrition which are (a) reliable and (b) do not generalize about dietary requirements. (The second stipulation guarantees the first, ordinarily.) When you have enough background to allow you to cooperate intelligently with a medical nutritionist, consult one. Don't reject this suggestion (or his advice) on the grounds that you're normal. Quite possibly, *that* is what needs changing. The doctor will monitor your mineral metabolism, your glucose tolerance, and your blood nutrients levels, your blood fats, but in the end the important questions will be: How are you sleeping?

Do you arise refreshed, feeling adequate to meet your responsibilities? Is your appetite good, your elimination adequate, your resistance to fatigue high? Are your attention and memory spans functioning as they should? What's happening with your nails, hair, skin, vision, digestion, muscle tone?

And as these subjective responses indicate that the proper pattern of nutrition for you, as an individual, has been achieved, you will realize that there is, in fact, an "I" in diet, a "U" in menu, that there are individual needs in nutrients which, satisfied, will help you to a higher plane of physical and intellectual functioning.

Appendix: Where to Seek Help

I HAVE COME to dread the aftermath of appearances in the media—radio, television, or newspapers—in which the topic was orthomolecular therapy for medical or psychiatric disorders, for the mail which cascades upon my staff is filled with desperation and frustration. The most frequent complaint: "I can't find a psychiatrist or a physician who doesn't look at me as if I were some kind of a nut, when I ask about nutritional treatments. They don't 'believe in' hypoglycemia, they laugh at orthomolecular and megavitamin treatment, or they tell me not to listen to pseudoscience on TV. Can you give the names of psychiatrists (or physicians) who are competent in this field? Preferably, in my neighborhood? I have a son. . . ." (Substitute wife, aged mother, schizophrenic daughter, alcoholic husband.)

It is then my turn to be frustrated. The lists of orthomolecular physicians and psychiatrists grow, month by month, but there are deserts which include some major cities, where no such specialist can be found; and imposing a geographical limitation, of course, compounds the difficulty of fulfilling the request.

There are, though, organizations in medicine, and some lay groups, who are able to refer you to such practitioners, as close as possible to you. In some cases, that will still mean a long journey, and one can only hope that the solution of the problem will be the reward for your effort; in many cases, it should be. When you write to any of the medical societies I am listing for you, remember to specify exactly the type of medical specialization you seek. It won't be profitable if you wind up with an orthomolecular practitioner who is a proctologist, when the problem is at the other end of the anatomy. And do remember to enclose a stamped, self-addressed, business-size envelope with your inquiry.

Medical societies whose membership includes orthomolecular physicians and orthomolecular psychiatrists, as well as dentists practicing nutrition, include:

> The International Academy of Nutrition and Preventive Medicine, P.O. Box 5832, Lincoln, Nebraska 68505.

> The Academy of Orthomolecular Psychiatry, (*see* Huxley Institute, *below*).

Other sources of information concerning practitioners include:

> Canadian Schizophrenia Foundation, 7375 Kingsway, Burnaby, British Columbia V3N 3B5, Canada.

> Huxley Institute for Biosocial Research, 900 N. Federal Hwy., Suite 330, Boca Raton, Florida 33432.

Index